Introduction to A & P + Integumentary System

Concise
Bulleted
Lecture Notes

By
Mostafa ElNaggar

Part 1/7
Human A&P Booklet with Clinical Implications

ISBN

***

Introduction to A & P + Integumentary System

Concise
Bulleted
Lecture Notes

By
Mostafa ElNaggar

Part 1/7
Human A&P Booklet with Clinical Implications

Contents

Preface

- This **concise** booklet offers a basic anatomical & physiological framework with clinical applications.
- It gives the **direct information** required to understand the subject and pass the test.
- It includes all the important information, in a **bulleted** form, with **simple language** and straight forward presentation.
- It is supported with **figures** and **diagrams** to clarify the important concepts.
- It allows you to study in small digestible bits of information, instead of using large, **boring textbook.**
- It is useful when teaching is in an **integrated** curriculum.
- You can go through it **very quickly**, and use it as a **quick revision** before the examination.
- You can select to read the material **relevant** to you and review it **several times** until you master it.
- It follows the standard **learning outcomes**.
- It could be supported with any **Atlas** of anatomy.
- It is designed to be taught in **one or two courses** of 3-6 credit hours.
- The booklet is published as one part or divided into **7 parts** to make it suitable for e-publishing.

Chapter 1: Introduction to A & P

Definitions:
Anatomy
- Study of the normal **structure** of the body
- Structure dictates the function

Physiology
- Study of the normal **function** of the body

Pathology
- Disturbed structure or function of the body → **Disease**

Section 1: General Organization of the body

Our body is organized as follows (Fig. 1), from smaller to larger levels:
- **Chemical** level:
  - Any matter is formed of **atoms**
  - Atoms combine to form **molecules**
- **Cellular** level:
  - Molecules form **cells**
  - Cells are the basic units of life (eg Nerve cells)
- **Tissue** level:
  - Cells form tissues (eg nerve cells form grey matter of the brain)
- **Organ** level: eg Grey and white matter form the brain organ
- **System** level: eg nervous system contains brain, spinal cord, nerves and ganglia.
- **Whole body (organism):** which contains all the systems

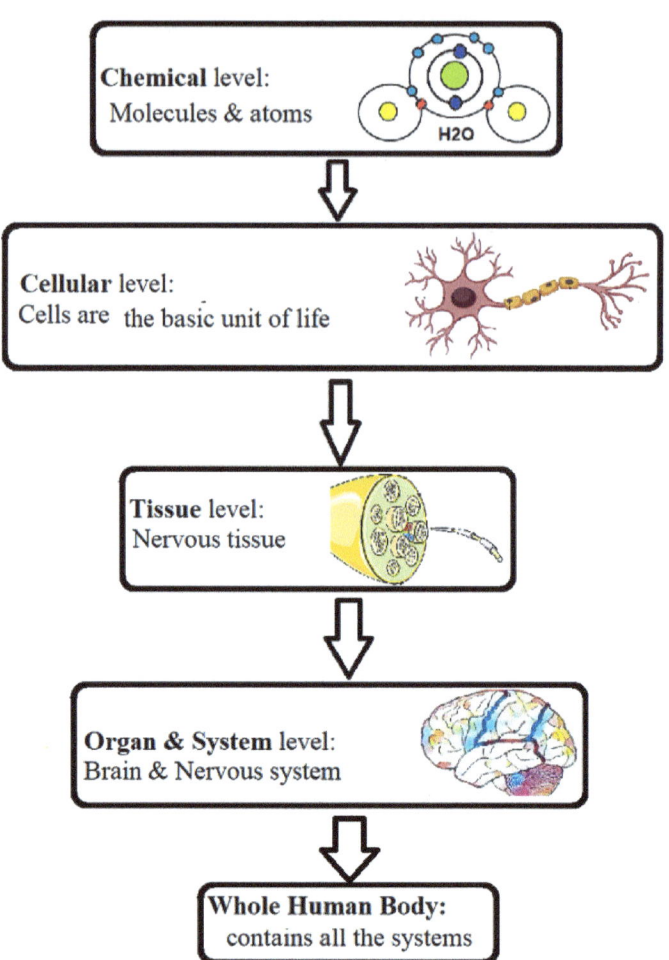

Figure 1: Levels of organization of the human body

Section 2: Chemical level of organization

Elements
- There are only 92 naturally occurring elements.
- Over 90% of the human body is composed of **4 elements**: carbon, nitrogen, oxygen & hydrogen.

Atoms
- An atom is **the smallest unit of an element** that still retains the chemical and physical properties of the element.
- Consists of **(Fig. 2) nucleus (Protons + Neutrons) & electrons** (in shells = orbits)
  - **Protons** carry a positive (+) charge,
  - **Neutrons** have no charge.
  - **Electrons** have a negative (−) charge.
- The **atomic number** = the number of **protons** in an atom.
- The **mass number** of an atom = the sum of **protons and neutrons** in an atom.

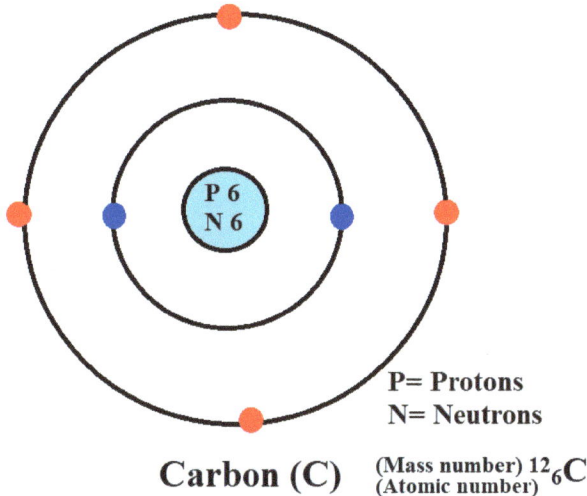

P= Protons
N= Neutrons

Carbon (C)   (Mass number) $^{12}_{6}$C
(Atomic number)

Figure 2: The carbon atom

- The **inner shell** can hold 2 electrons.
- The next **shell** can hold 8 electrons.
- An atom is most **stable** when the outermost shell has 8 electrons. (or 2 electrons in case of hydrogen and helium, having one shell)
- An atom → becomes an **ion** when it gains or loses electrons
  - when it gains electrons → it becomes a **negative** ion (-).
  - when it loses electrons → it becomes a **positive** ion (+).

Molecules:

- Atoms unite together to form molecules
- The large molecules (**macromolecules**) of the body are: proteins, carbohydrates, fats, and nucleic acids (as DNA).

Isotopes
- Are elements (atoms) with different number of **neutrons** → therefore they have different mass number (weight).
- Example: **Carbon** has 3 isotopes
  - $^{12}_{6}C$ has 6 neutrons
  - $^{13}_{6}C$ has 7 neutrons
  - $^{14}_{6}C$* has 8 neutrons, is **radioactive**, its radiation could be detected by **Geiger counter**

Biological & medical use of isotopes:
- **Radioactive iodine tracer** can be absorbed by the thyroid gland → to detect cancer thyroid cells.
- **Killing cancer cells**: for treatment of cancer
- **Sterilizing** medical products

Electron shells of the atom:
- **Electron Shells**: are the orbits for the electrons around the nucleus of an atom **(Fig. 3)**.
  - First shell: is the nearest to the nucleus. It can hold 2 electrons.
  - Second shell: can hold 8 electrons.
  - Third shell: can hold 8 electrons.
- **Valence shell** is the outermost shell of the atom.

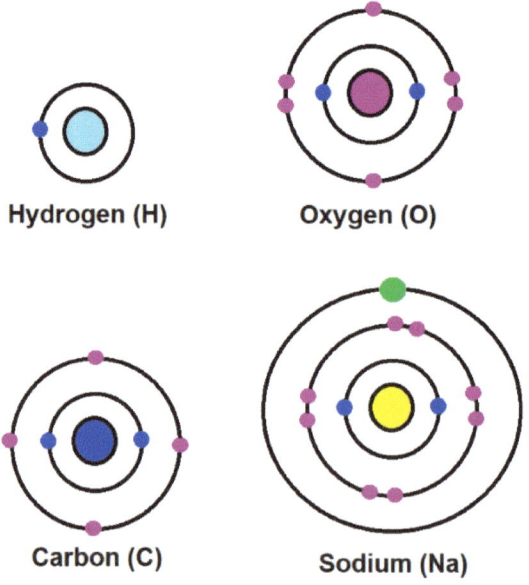

Hydrogen (H)   Oxygen (O)

Carbon (C)   Sodium (Na)

Figure 3: Electron shells of common elements

Valence (Valency)
- **The number of bonds** an atom forms.
- **The number of electrons required** to be lost or gained to achieve a stable **outermost shell.**
- Valence lies between 1 and 7

Types of chemical bonds
1) Ionic bonds
- **Ions** **loose or gain** one or more valence **electrons** (from the outer shell).
- Loosing electron → gives **positive** ion (**cation**), as **Na⁺**
- Gaining electron → gives **negative** ion (**anion**), as **Cl⁻**
- Positive and negative ions are attracted together.
- **Na** can give its valence electron to the Cl→ Na Cl (**Fig. 4**).
- **Electrolytes** are ions in solution
  - **Cations** (⁺): Na⁺, K⁺, Ca⁺⁺, Mg⁺⁺, H⁺
  - **Anions** (⁻): Cl⁻, HCO³⁻, PO⁴⁻

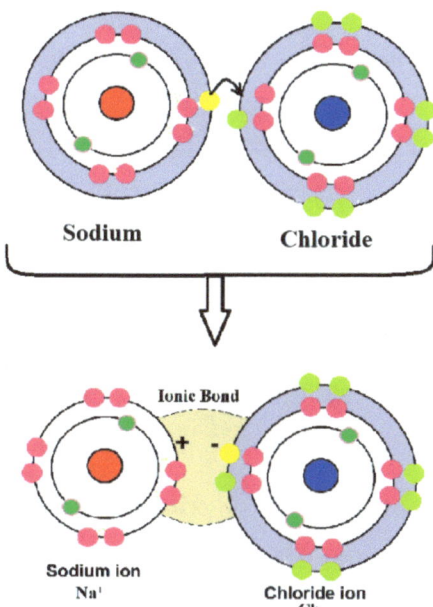

Figure 4: Ionic bond between Na⁺ and Cl⁻ ions forming sodium chloride

2) Covalent bonds
- Atoms **share outer electrons**, not gaining or loosing (**Fig. 5**).
- **Single** covalent bond: sharing one pair of electrons

- **Double** covalent bond: sharing two pairs of electrons
- **Triple** covalent bond: sharing three pairs of electrons

Polar & non-polar Covalent bond

- **Polar:** Share electrons **unequally**
    - One of the elements keeps the electrons for a longer time.
    - Such element will be **electronegative**
- **non-polar:** atoms share electrons **equally**
- Electronegative elements arranged from least to greatest:
C < N < O < F
- Water (**H_2O**) forms **polar** covalent bonds
- Electrons spend most of their time with the **electronegative oxygen**, because it has a larger atom.

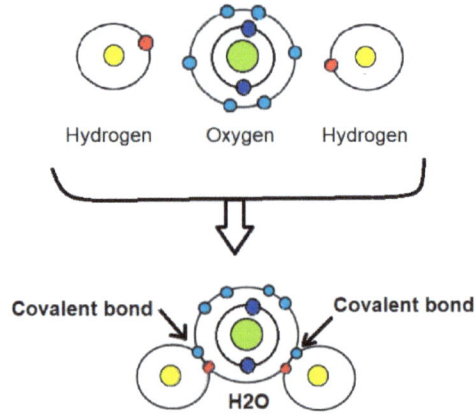

Figure 5: Covalent bonds of water (H_2O)

Structural formulas use straight lines to show the **covalent bonds** between atoms. Each **line** represents a pair of shared electrons.
Molecular formulas indicate the **number** of each atom making up a molecule.

- **Example**
    - Structural formula   Molecular formula
        Cl—Cl Cl_2
        O=C=O CO_2

3) Hydrogen bonds

- They are **weak** bonds present between **parts of water molecules (Fig. 6)**.
- Formed by attraction between positive and negative parts of water molecules

- not sharing electrons (as in covalent bond)
- not losing or gaining of electrons (as in ionic bond).
- Are represented by dotted lines.
- Function
  - Formation of the **surface tension**.
  - Formation of the **three dimensional shape** of large molecules.
  - Causing **cohesion** (water attracted to water) and **adhesion** (water attracted to other molecule).

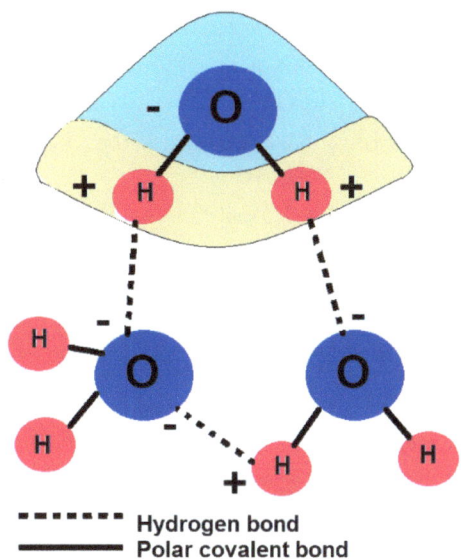

Figure 6: Hydrogen bonds between water molecules

- **Solvent** = dissolving medium. It is usually liquid (as water).
- **Solutes** = substances in smaller amounts, dissolved in the solvent.

Water as a solvent

- Water is a **solvent** for **ionized (polar)** substances, due to its polar covalent bonds
- **Solutes** are divided into:
  - **Hydrophilic**: are charged (have polar covalent bonds) and are soluble in water.
    - Example: in NaCl, water surrounds and separates the ions of **Na$^+$ and Cl$^-$** (this is called **hydrolysis)**
  - **Hydrophobic**: have non-polar covalent bonds and are not water soluble
- have high **specific heat capacity** (is the amount of heat needed to change temperature by 1°C)
  - Insulates the body from extreme heat & extreme cold

- high **heat of vapor** (the amount of energy needed to turn water into steam)
  - Sweating cools the body rapidly and effectively
- Water molecules dissociate to form equal numbers of hydrogen ions (H^+) and hydroxide ions (OH^-):
  - ✓ **$H-O-H \rightarrow H^+ + OH^-$**
- **Acids** dissociate in water, releasing **(H+)** (are a **proton donors**)
  - ✓ For example **HCl**, dissociates to **H^+ & Cl^-**
  - ✓ **$HCl \rightarrow H^+ + Cl^-$**
- **Bases** either take up **(H+)** or release **(OH−)**
  - sodium hydroxide (NaOH), which dissociates into: **Na^+ & OH^-**
  - **$NaOH \rightarrow Na^+ + OH^-$**
- When an acid and a base are combined, the reaction produces **salt** and water.
  - For example: **$HCl + NaOH \rightarrow NaCl + H_2O$**

pH & Buffers
pH= minus (-) log of **H^+ ion** concentration
•pH 7.0 = 1/10,000,000 ions/ liter
The pH scale ranges from 0 to 14
  - pH above 7 is basic (alkaline)
  - pH below 7 is acidic
- As we move toward a lower pH, each unit has 10 times the acidity of the previous unit.
  - Example: pH 2 (0.01 moles/liter) has 100 times *more* H+ than a solution of pH 4 (0.0001 moles/liter)
- as pH *decreases,* H+ concentration exponentially *increases.*
- **Example**: A solution containing **0.00001 moles per liter** of free hydrogen ions = **1×10^{-5} moles per liter = pH 5**.
- Normal pH of **blood** = 7.4 (range 7.35 – 7.45)
  - **Acidosis:** pH below 7.35
  - **Alkalosis** pH above 7.45
- Mechanisms to prevent pH changes:
  1. Buffers in blood
  2. Respiratory system
  3. Urinary system

Buffers:
- **Buffers** consist of a weak acid + corresponding weak base.
- They help to **stabilize** pH within normal & prevent excess acid or base **(Fig. 7)**.

12

- Important buffers in the body are:
    - **Carbonic acid/ bicarbonate** buffer
    - Phosphate buffer
    - Protein buffer

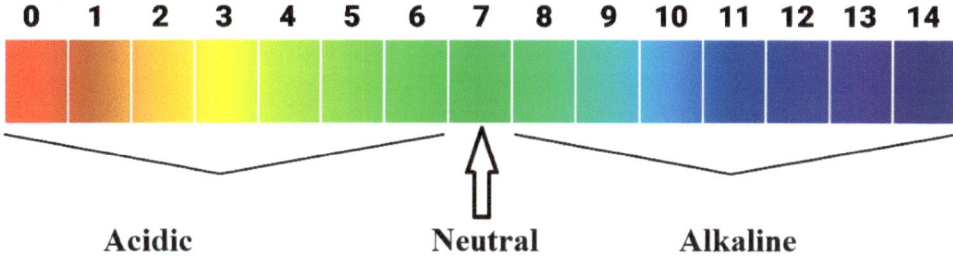

Figure 7: pH scale

How bicarbonate buffer system works?
- The **weak acid** is carbonic acid (H_2CO_3). It dissociates reversibly, $\rightarrow$ releasing, bicarbonate ions (HCO_3^-) **(weak base)** and protons (H^+):
$$H_2CO_3 \longleftrightarrow HCO_3^- + H^+$$
- If blood pH raises (more **alkaline**) $\rightarrow$ the equilibrium shifts to the right $\rightarrow$ more carbonic acid dissociates giving $H^+\rightarrow$ neutralizes OH^-
- If blood pH drops (more **acidic**) $\rightarrow$ the equilibrium shifts to the left $\rightarrow$ as more bicarbonate ions bind with H^+.

Biochemistry
- It is the study of the chemical composition of **living matter**.
- It lies into 2 classes:
    - Organic compounds
    - Inorganic compounds.

Organic compounds contain **carbon**, which is <u>**characterized by:**</u>
- It is **electro-neutral**, meaning it never loses or gains electrons, but shares electrons.
- It can form **4 covalent bonds**.
- Carbon atoms can unite with each other to form **polymer**
    - Polymers are **formed** by dehydration (**covalent bond**) **(Fig. 8)**
    - Polymers are **decomposed** by rehydration (hydrolysis)

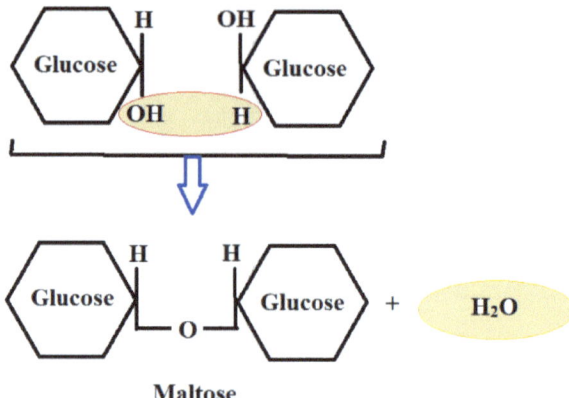

Figure 8: Covalent bonds made by dehydration to form disaccharide

Types of organic compounds:
1. carbohydrates
2. fats
3. proteins
4. nucleic acids

I] Carbohydrates
- They are the source of energy.
- They are formed of monosaccharides.

Monosaccharides:
- are monomeric building blocks
- soluble in water
- single chain of 3-7 carbon atoms
- They have C: H: O in the ratio 1:2:1
- Their general formula is: $(CH_2O)_n$
- They are named according to the number of the carbon atoms:
    - **pentose** (5-carbon sugars) as deoxyribose (is part of DNA)
    - **Hexose** (6-carbon sugars) as glucose & its isomers galactose and fructose.

Disaccharides:
- Are two monosaccharides joined by dehydration (covalent bond)
    $2 C_6H_{12}O_6 \rightarrow C_{12}H_{22}O_{11}+H_2O$
- glucose + fructose $\rightarrow$ sucrose + water
- Important disaccharides in the body:
    - **Sucrose**= glucose + fructose
    - **Lactose**= glucose + galactose

14

– **Maltose**= glucose + glucose

Polysaccharides
- are large insoluble **polymers**
- Examples
    - **Starch**: in plants, is branched.
    - **Glycogen**: in animals (skeletal muscles & liver), is highly branched
    - **Cellulose**: is found in plant cell walls. Humans cannot digest it because they lack the enzyme **cellulase**.

II| Lipids
- They contain C, H, & O (proportion of O is much lower).
- May contain phosphorus.
- Lipids include triglycerides, phospholipids & steroids

1) Triglycerides
- They are known as **fats** when solid or **oils** when liquid.
- **Fats** are of animal origin (e.g. lard and butter)
- **Oils** are of plant origin (e.g. corn oil and soybean oil)
- They provide the most efficient store of energy.
- They are composed of **3 fatty acids** + **glycerol**, in a 3: 1 ratio **(Fig. 9)**
- **Oils** are **liquid** because of their unsaturated fatty acids.
- **Unsaturated fatty acid**: has double bond between carbon atoms **(Fig. 9)**.
- **Hydrogenation** of vegetable oils can convert them to **margarine**
- diet high in saturated fats and cholesterol → can cause accumulation of fatty material inside the wall of blood vessels → **atherosclerosis** → reducing blood flow

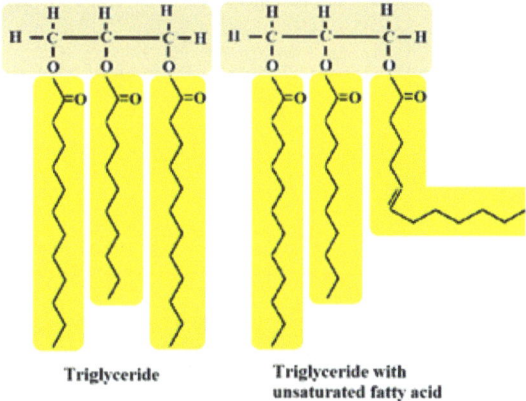

Triglyceride

Triglyceride with unsaturated fatty acid

Figure 9: Chemical structure of Triglyceride

- **Fatty acids** are linear hydrocarbon chains (H & C) with an organic acid group (-COOH) at one end.
  - They are **non-polar** molecules which do not mix with water.
- **Glycerol** is a modified simple sugar (sugar alcohol).

Emulsification: is mixing of fat with water
- **Emulsifiers** are substances which cause fats to mix with water.
  - They contain molecules with a nonpolar end and a polar end.
  - The molecules position themselves around an oil droplet so that their **polar ends project out**.
  - **Soaps and detergents** can remove fats and oils from dirty clothes or dishes.
  - **Bile** is the emulsifier produced by the liver, stored in the gallbladder, and released when we eat a fatty meal.

2) Phospholipids

- Consists of Glycerol + 2 fatty acids + phosphate group + nitrogen-containing group **(Fig. 10)**
- They form the main component of the cell membrane.

It has **two parts**
- **Polar head**: Glycerol + phosphate group + nitrogen-containing group
- **Non polar tail**: 2 fatty acids

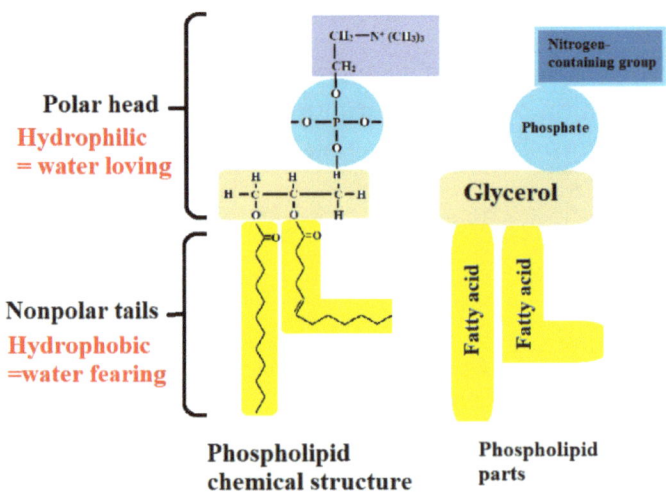

Figure 10: Structure of phospholipid

3) Steroids

- Formed of 4 hydrocarbon rings **(Fig. 11)**
- Example: **cholesterol** which is found in
  - cell membrane
  - vitamin D
  - steroid hormones & bile salts
- Cholesterol is the precursor of some hormones:
  - **testosterone**
  - **estrogens**

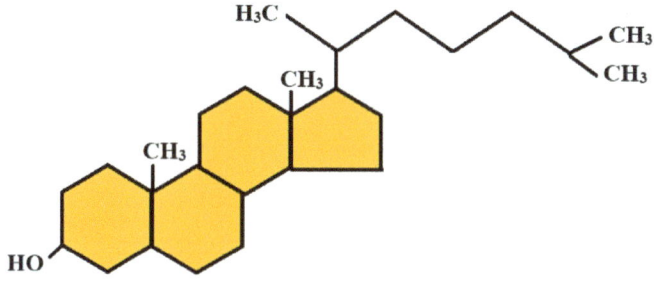

Figure 11: Steroid structure

<u>Eicosanoids</u>
- are derived from **arachidonic acid** (fatty acid with 20-carbon)
- are found in all cell membranes
- Example: **prostaglandins** which play a role in inflammation
  - They are blocked by **NSAIDs** (nonsteroidal anti-inflammatory drugs; e.g., ibuprofen)

III] Proteins

- **Amino acids (AA)**
  - Form the building units of **proteins**
  - There are 20 types of AA.
  - All AA contain C, O, H, & N, and 2 of them contain sulfur.
  - all AA have **2 functional groups** (**& R group**)
  - The 2 functional groups are:
    - ✓ **amine group** (-NH$_2$): act as a base (proton acceptor)
    - ✓ **acid group** (-COOH): act as an acid (proton donor).
  - **R group** is unique for each AA
  - Each AA can act as base or acid.

- **Proteins**:
  - Are long chain of AA connected with peptide bonds

- **Peptide bond**: is a dehydration synthesis linking the acid end of one AA to the amine end of the next **(Fig. 12)**.
- Dipeptide: 2 AA
- Tripeptide 3 AA
- **Polypeptide**: 10 or more AA
- **Proteins**: are polypeptides containing more than 50 AA
- **Macromolecules**: containing from 100 to over 10,000 AA.

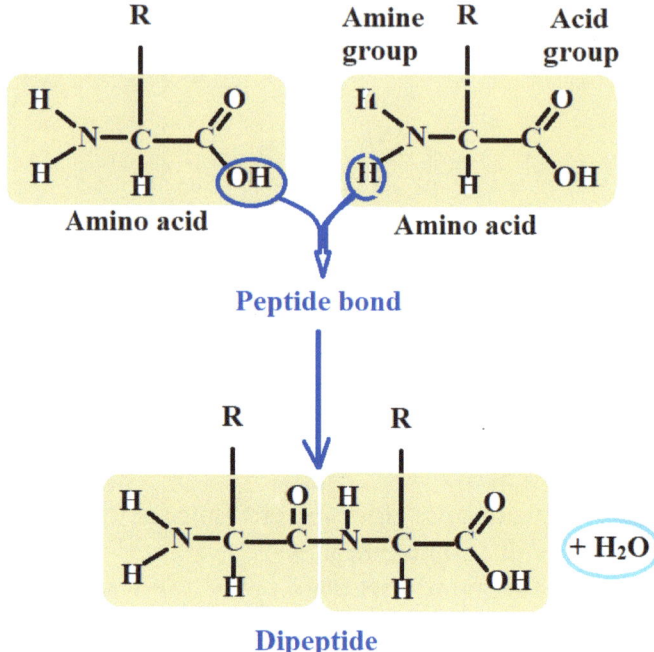

Figure 12: Structure of amino acid and peptide bond

Structural levels of proteins

- **Primary**: is the **linear** sequence of AA in the polypeptide chain
- **Secondary**: The primary chain forms **spirals** (α-helices) and **sheets** (β-sheets).
- **Tertiary**: secondary structures are **folded up** to form a compact **globular** molecule.
- **Quaternary**: **Two or more polypeptide chains**, each with its own tertiary structure, combine to form a **functional** protein.

Types of proteins

Fibrous proteins = **structural** proteins

- Are very stable, insoluble in water
- Provide mechanical support and strength to the tissues.

- Example:
  - **collagen** is made of helical **tropocollagen** molecules
  - **contractile proteins**

<u>Globular</u> proteins = **functional** proteins
- Are compact, spherical, have at least tertiary structure, water soluble, chemically active, biologically functional
- Include enzymes.

Protein denaturation
- Protein structure is maintained by weak hydrogen bonds, which are fragile and could be easily broken (by temp, pH)
- **Denatured protein:** unfolded protein that loses its specific three-dimensional shape → disruption of the active site → loss of function of the protein.
- Extreme cases are irreversible, like **egg white boiling**.

Enzymes
- **Enzymes** are globular proteins that act as biological catalysts.
- **Catalysts** are substances that accelerate the rate of reactions (up to billion times) but are not used up or changed in those reactions.

Characteristics of enzymes
- The **holoenzyme** consists of 2 parts
  - **Apo enzyme** (the protein part)
  - **Cofactor**: which may be
    - metal element as cupper or iron,
    - organic molecule called **coenzyme**, mostly derived from vitamin B complex).
- Enzymes bind to specific molecules.
- **Substrate:** is the substance on which an enzyme acts.

- **Enzyme action**
  - Every reaction requires **activation energy.**
  - Enzymes decrease the activation energy required.
  - Three basic steps **(Fig. 13)**
    1. **Substrate** binds temporarily to the **enzyme active site** → forming an **enzyme-substrate complex** →
    2. undergoes internal rearrangements that form the **product**
    3. The enzyme releases the product & returns to its original shape.

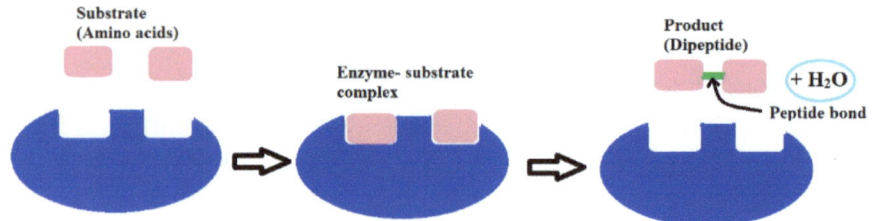

Figure 13: Enzyme action

Prion (protein infectious particle) → causes transmissible **spongiform encephalopathies** (**TSEs**).

- In humans it causes **Creutzfeldt-Jakob disease**.
- Nerve cells contain **normal type of prion** protein, its function is unknown.
- Abnormal prions → cause nervous system destruction, including
  - ✓ Alzheimer's disease
  - ✓ Parkinson's disease
  - ✓ amyotrophic lateral sclerosis

IV] Nucleic acids
- 2 major classes: DNA & RNA

DNA
- Deoxyribonucleic acid
- Contains Deoxyribose Sugar
- Double strand coiled into a double helix
- Contain Adenine (A), guanine (G), cytosine (C), thymine (T)
- is found in the nucleus
- Forms the genome of the cell
- Has 2 roles:
  - It **replicates** (reproduces) itself before the cell divides.
  - It provides the basic instructions for **building proteins**
- DNA fingerprinting → can help solve forensic problems

RNA
- Ribonucleic acid
- Sugar: Ribose
- Single strand, straight or folded
- Contains Adenine (A), uracil (U), guanine (G), cytosine (C)
- U replaces T of DNA.
- Function: carries out the orders of DNA for **protein synthesis**.

- **3 major types** of RNA according to size and shape
  - messenger **mRNA**
  - ribosomal **rRNA**
  - transfer **tRNA**

Nucleotides:
- Are the structural units of nucleic acids
- Each nucleotide consists of 3 components
  - **base** that contains nitrogen
  - **pentose sugar**
  - **phosphate** group
- There are 5 **bases** that belong to 2 groups:

Purines: larger, with two-ring bases
- Adenine (A)
- Guanine (G)

Pyrimidines: smaller, with single-ring base
- cytosine (C)
- thymine (T)
- uracil (U)

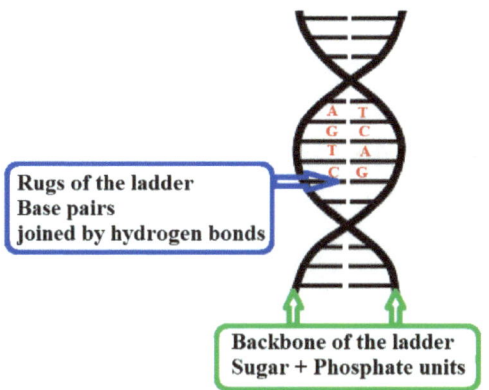

Rugs of the ladder
Base pairs
joined by hydrogen bonds

Backbone of the ladder
Sugar + Phosphate units

Figure 14: Structure of DNA

Structure of DNA
- DNA is a long, coiled, spiral double chain of **nucleotides helix** (sugar + phosphate) connected by **rugs** of bases (A, T, G, C)
- The bases bind to each other by hydrogen bonds, in a **complementary** specific way (**base-pairing**) (Fig. 14)

How?
- **A** binds to **T**.
- **G** binds to **C**.

Example:
- **AGTC** on one DNA strand will bind to **TCAG** (a complementary base sequence) on the other strand.

Adenosine triphosphate (ATP)
- It stores energy released from glucose in high energy bonds
- **Structure**: ATP = adenine + sugar (ribose) + Phosphate (P) □ P □ P **(Fig. 15)**
- Phosphate groups are attached by **high energy** phosphate bonds (□).
- **Phosphorylation:** is the transfer of the terminal phosphate group from ATP to another molecule by an enzyme
  - **ATP** = adenine + sugar (ribose) + Phosphate (P) □ P □ P
  - **ATP** + H_2O → **ADP** + P_i (inorganic phosphate) + energy
  - **ADP** + H_2O → **AMP** + P_i (inorganic phosphate) + energy

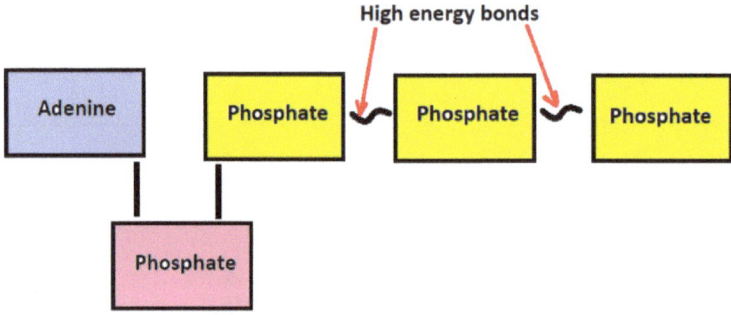

Figure 15: Structure of ATP

Section 3: Cell structure & function

- Cells are the basic structural & functional units of life.

Basic Cell Functions

1. Obtaining **food (nutrients) and O^2** from the environment.
2. **Eliminating carbon dioxide** (CO^2) and wastes.
3. Using nutrients and O2 to **provide energy**
   Food + O^2 → CO^2 + H^2O + energy
4. **Synthesizing proteins** for growth, and for cell functions.
5. **Exchange** of materials with the surrounding environment.
6. **Moving materials** internally
7. **Respond** to changes in the surrounding.
8. **Reproduction** (Except nerve and muscle cells)
   - Brain, and heart attacks, can be devastating.

Cell structure
- All cells have **three regions (Fig. 16):**
   - Cytoplasm
   - Plasma membrane
   - Nucleus (except RBC)

I. Cytoplasm
   - The cytoplasm contains the following **organelles**:
      - Endoplasmic reticulum
      - Golgi complex
      - secretory vesicles
      - lysosomes
      - mitochondria
      - microtubules & microfilaments

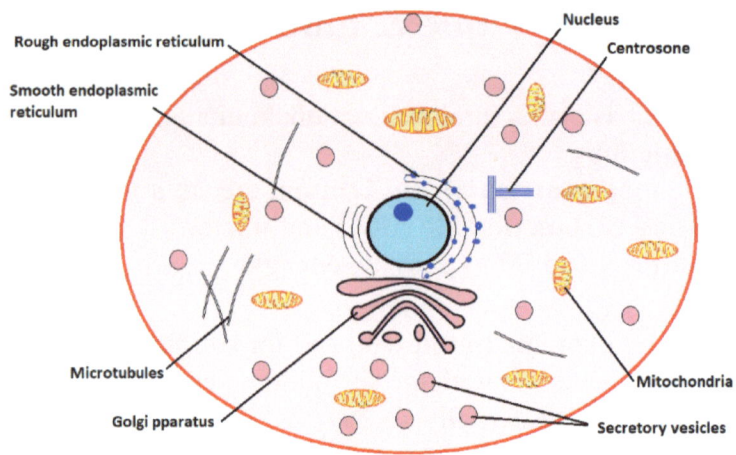

Figure 16: The structure of the cell

Endoplasmic Reticulum (ER)
- Is a membrane system
- Formed of **Two types**: rough and smooth **(Fig. 17)**
    - **rough ER:** formed of stacks of flat **sacs**
    - **smooth ER:** formed of meshwork of **tubules**

The rough ER (RER)
- Function: synthesizes proteins for secretion
- Its outer surface contains **attached ribosomes (rRNA)**
- **rRNA** → synthesizes and releases **new proteins** into the **ER lumen**, → **for export**

<u>**free ribosomes**</u> → synthesize proteins for use within the cell.

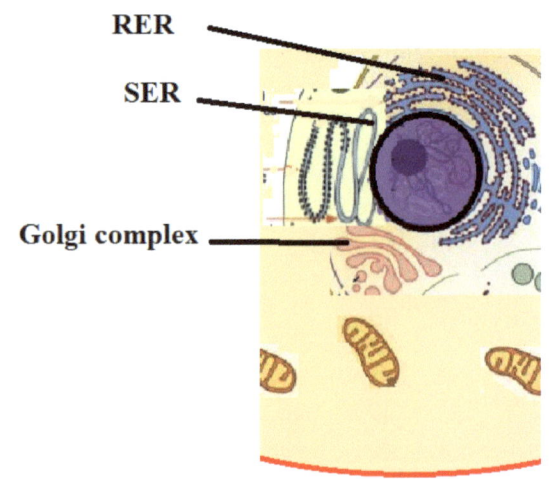

Figure 17: Endoplasmic reticulum (ER)

The smooth ER (SER)
- Function: **packaging** of new proteins (formed in rough RE) in **transport vesicles** → move them to the **Golgi complex**.

Golgi Complex
- consists of a stack of **flattened, curved sacs (Fig. 18)**
- have dilated, or bulging, edges
- Are numerous in highly specialized cells, for protein secretion.
- When a **transport vesicle** reaches a **Golgi stack** → **it** fuses with its sac → release its content to the interior of the sac → travels through the layers of the Golgi stacks → to the outermost sacs near the **plasma membrane** → **exocytosis**.

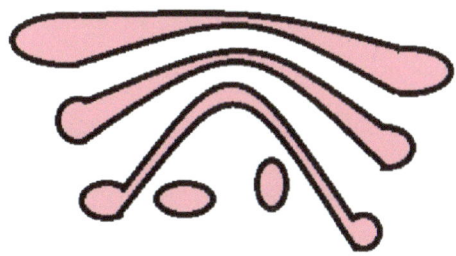

Figure 18: Golgi complex

Function of Golgi complex
1. **Sorting and directing** the finished products to their final destinations (exocytosis or internal use)
2. **Processing** the raw materials → into finished product → secretion by **exocytosis (Fig. 19)**
- **Example**: secretion of protein hormones, and digestive enzymes

Endocytosis:
- form endocytotic pouch → is pinched inward to form **vesicle**
- Endocytosis can be accomplished in three ways:
1. *Pinocytosis: Cell drinking*
2. *Phagocytosis: Cell eating* **(Fig. 19)**
3. *Receptor-mediated endocytosis:* Binding of a specific molecule (as a protein) to a surface specific **membrane receptor**.
   - ✓ **Examples:** Cholesterol complexes, vitamin B12, insulin hormone, iron, *some viruses*.

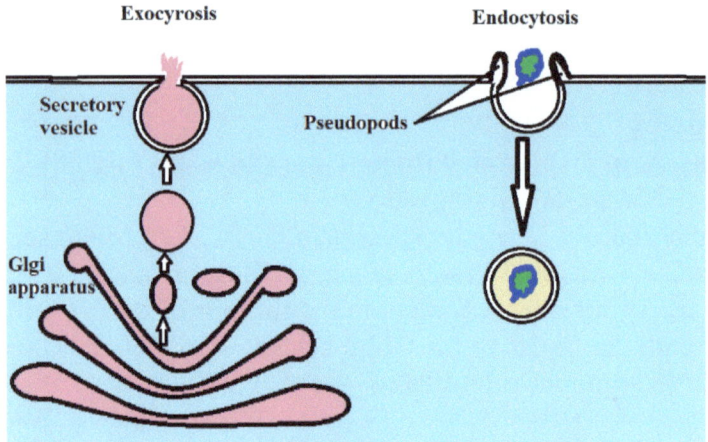

Figure 19: Exocytosis- Endocytosis

Lysosomes
- **Lysosomes** are small, membranous vesicles that break down organic molecules (lys = breakdown; some = body).
- Contain **hydrolytic enzymes** → digest the following:
  - **phagocytosed materials**.
  - **Old organelles**.
- Some individuals **lack one or more of the lysosomal enzymes** → accumulation of material inside the lysosomes (=*storage diseases*)
  - *example:* **Tay-Sachs disease,** which is characterized by abnormal accumulation of complex molecules in nerve cells → leading to **progressive nervous-system degeneration**.

Peroxisomes
- **Peroxisomes** are membranous vesicles that produce and decompose **hydrogen peroxide (H_2O_2)**
- Have **oxidative Enzymes**.
- Detoxify various wastes produced or foreign toxic compounds, such as **alcohol**.
- They **form H_2O_2** from molecular O_2.
- Decomposes potent H_2O_2 → into harmless $H_2O + O_2$.

Mitochondria
- are the "**power plants**" of the cell
- They extract energy from food nutrients → transform it into ATP.
- are rod-shaped or oval structures.

- Have double membrane—a **smooth outer membrane**, and an **inner membrane** that forms **shelves** called **cristae (Fig. 20)**
- The **matrix** have enzymes that start energy extraction from food.
- The **cristae** contain enzymes that convert energy in food into ATP

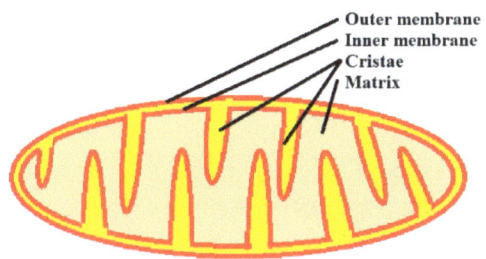

Figure 20: Mitochondria

Cytoskeleton
- Are bones & muscles of the cell
- Three distinct elements: **microtubules**, microfilaments (**actin** and **myosin** filaments), and **intermediate** filaments

(1) *microtubules*
- Long, slender, hollow **tubes**
- composed of globular protein called **tubulin**
- They can **assemble and disassemble**.

Function:
1. **Move** the organelles, by assembling and disassembling.
2. transport of secretory **vesicles**
3. maintain the **shape** of cells, such as nerve cells
4. coordinate complex cell movements
5. Form the main component of **cilia**, **flagella** and **mitotic spindle** (during cell division).

Cilia
- are hair like protrusions found on the surface of a ciliated cell (as respiratory epithelium).
- **beat** in a given direction
- Examples
  - The **respiratory** cilia keep foreign particles out
  - In the female **oviduct**, for transport of the egg (ovum)

Flagella
- long, whip like appendages
- Example: human **sperms**
- It enables the sperm to move & fertilize the female ovum.

2) filaments
- **Actin** filaments
  - − are long, thin fibers, present in bundles.
  - − They can **assemble and disassemble**.
  - − *Present in the* **Microvilli** (in the intestines).
- **Myosin** filaments
  - − Associated with movements, such as in **muscle** cells.

3) Intermediate filaments
- Are tough and resist **stress**
- Present in cell-to-cell junctions.
- join skin cells of the **epidermis**.

II. Plasma Membrane
- **Structure**: **Phospholipid bilayer (Fig. 21)** with small amounts of
  - − **cholesterol**
  - − **proteins**
  - − **Carbohydrate**

- Let's build up the plasma membrane one block after another.

First block: Phospholipid bilayer
have a **polar head**
- containing a negatively charged phosphate group
- **is hydrophilic** "water loving" it can interact with water molecules, which are also polar

2 **nonpolar tails** (electrically neutral) fatty acid chains
- **is hydrophobic** "water fearing"

- The bilayer have:
  - − Outer surface exposed to **ECF**,
  - − inner surface in contact with the intracellular fluid (**ICF**).

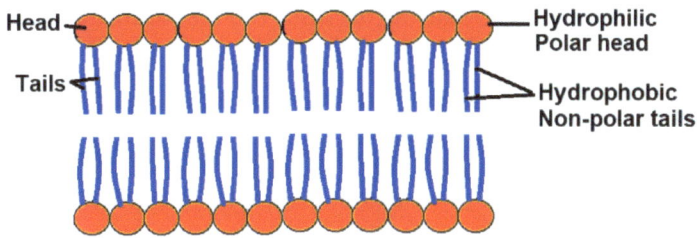

Figure 21: Phospholipid bilayer of the plasma membrane

- The **Phospholipid bilayer** appears with **electron microscope** as **trilaminar membrane**
    - Two dark lines (the polar heads)
    - separated by a light middle layer (the hydrophobic tails).
- **Fluid mosaic model**: The **phospholipids** are not rigid, they are constantly moving, exchanging places millions of times every second.
    - This enables many membrane proteins to float freely like "icebergs".

Functions of the lipid bilayer
- Its hydrophobic interior is a **barrier** to passage of water soluble substances.
- It is responsible for the **fluidity** of the membrane.

<u>Cholesterol</u>
- Is present between the phospholipid molecules **(Fig. 22)**.
- It gives the membrane its **fluidity** and **stability**, enabling the **cell to change shape**.

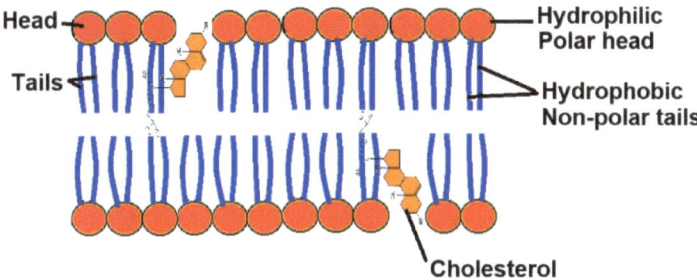

Figure 22: Phospholipid bilayer with cholesterol

<u>Second block: proteins</u>
- 2 types **(Fig. 23)**

– **Integral**: extend throughout the entire thickness of the membrane
– **Peripheral**: present at the outer or inner surface of the membrane

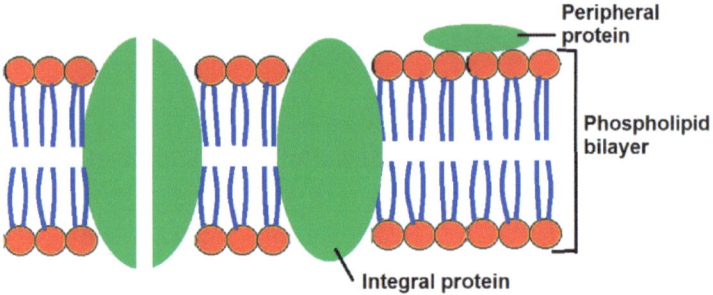

Figure 23: Phospholipid plasma membrane with proteins

Functions of the membrane proteins
- Form water-filled pathways (**channels**)
- Form **carrier** (transport) molecules
- **Docking** acceptors for secretory vesicles before exocytosis.
- Form **cell adhesion** molecules (CAMs).
- **Receptor** sites e.g. for **water-soluble hormones**, as thyroid stimulating hormone (TSH)
- **Membrane-bound enzymes,** For example, enzymes of **skeletal muscle** cells that destroy ACh.
- **Recognize "self"** (cells of the same type) in conjunction with carbohydrates.

Third block: carbohydrates
- Short carbohydrate chains (**Fig. 24**)
- protrude from the outer surface of the membrane
- Attached to the membrane proteins.
- **Function: "self-recognition"** and cell-to-cell interactions.

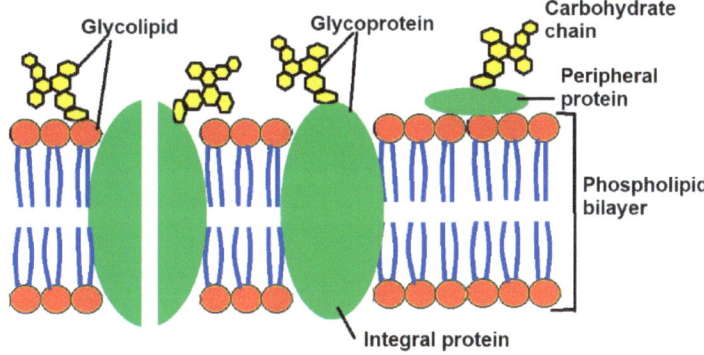

Figure 24: Phospholipid plasma membrane with proteins & carbohydrates

Material transport across the Plasma Membrane

<u>Simple Diffusion</u>

Example: Diffusion through membrane **(Fig. 25)**

Factors which affect the rate of diffusion **(Fick's Law** of Diffusion):

- **Concentration** gradient across the membrane
- **Area** of the membrane
- **Molecular weight** of the substance:
  - O^2 and CO^2 diffuse rapidly
- **Permeability** of the membrane to the substance
- The **distance** of diffusion
- **Temperature**: Kinetic energy increases with temperature

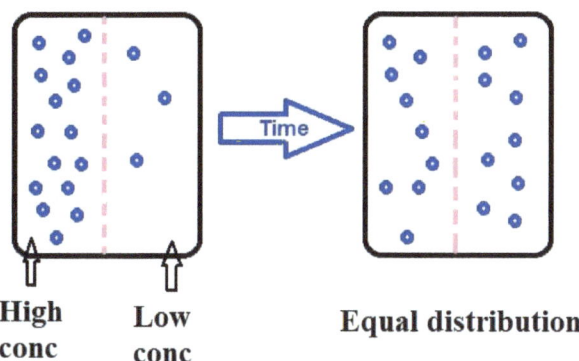

Figure 25: Diffusion through membrane

<u>Osmosis</u>

- Osmosis is **diffusion of water** through the semi-permeable membrane down concentration gradient **(Fig. 26)**.

- It occurs when the **solute is unable to move** down its concentration gradient.
- Osmosis stops when **equilibrium** is reached.
- **Osmotic pressure (the pulling force)** of a solution is the measure of tendency of a solution to pull water into it

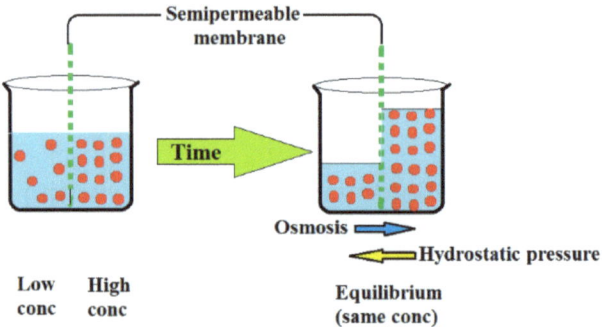

Figure 26: Movement of water by osmosis

Tonicity

- **Tonicity** (tono = tension) is the ability of a solution to **change the shape of the cells** by changing the cells' internal water volume **(Fig. 27)**.

Tonicity has 3 states:

- **Isotonic solution**: have the same concentrations of the solutes inside the cells
    - Example: **0.9% saline** or **5% glucose**.
- **Hypotonic solutions** are more dilute than cells.
    - Cells swell rapidly as water enters into them → they finally **burst**.
    - Example: **distilled water**.
- **Hypertonic solutions** have a higher concentration than the cell
    - Cells lose water → **crenate**.
    - Example: **strong saline** solution.

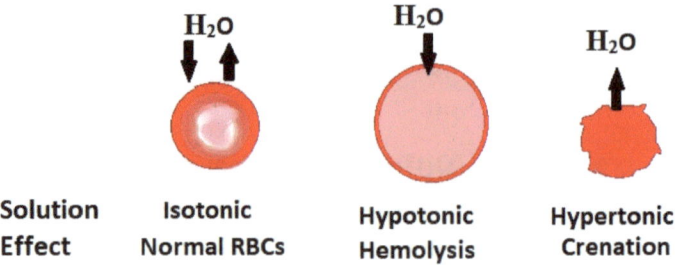

Figure 27: Osmosis and tonicity of RBCs

Types of transport through the plasma membrane (Fig. 28)
1] Passive transport:
- occurs according to concentration gradient or electric gradient (electrochemical gradient)
- No ATP is needed
- simple diffusion of **fat soluble substances**
  - Examples: O_2, CO_2, fatty acids. They ae fat soluble and pass directly through the plasma membrane.
- Simple diffusion of **water soluble substances**
  - Occur through water filled **channels**

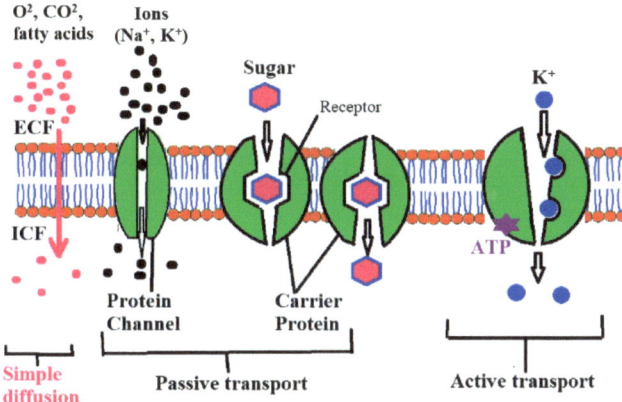

Figure 28: Types of membrane transport

2] Facilitated transport:
- Is a **passive transport, carrier mediated**
- doesn't need ATP
- Uses **channel protein** = protein carrier **changing its shape**.
- Example: **thyroid** gland cells have carriers for iodine.

- **Symport of glucose**
  - Na^+ K^+ pump creates concentration gradient with high Na^+ outside. Na^+ tends to enter the cell taking with it glucose, using the **symport carrier protein**
  - Example: **Na^+ and glucose** cotransport in intestinal epithelial cells (**Fig. 29**).

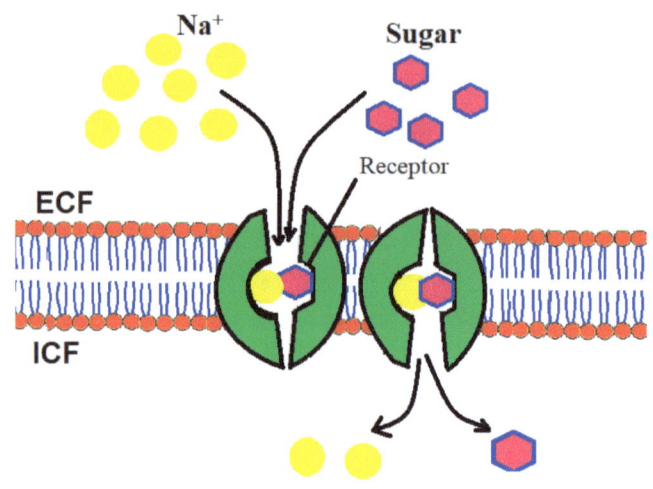

Figure 29: Sodium- glucose symport

<u>3] **Active transport**</u>:
- Requires energy (ATP) to transport the molecule **uphill** (from low concentration to high concentration).
- It uses **protein pump**
- Example: **Na^+/K^+ ATPase pump (Fig. 30)** found in the plasma membrane of all cells.

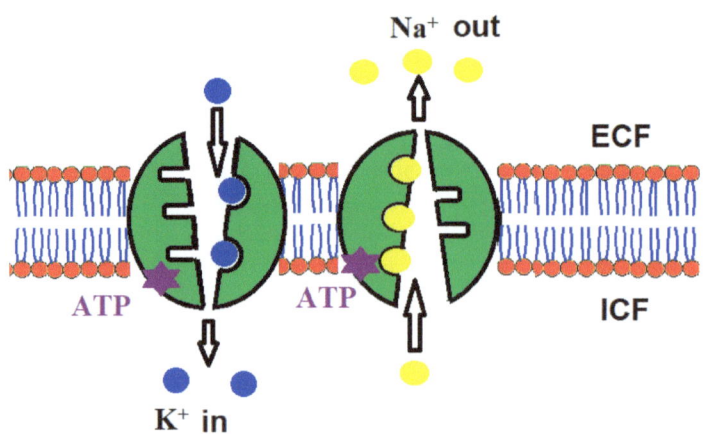

Figure 30: Sodium potassium pump

4] Vesicular transport
Was described with the cytoplasm

Cystic fibrosis (CF)
- Is the most common fatal genetic disease in US
- It affects 1 in every 2000 Caucasian children.
- Affects the following:
    - **Respiratory airways**: → production of **thick, sticky mucus**, → **fibrotic** lung, → becomes harder to inflate.
    - The **pancreatic duct**: → plugged with **thick mucus** → Fluid-filled **pancreatic cysts**,
- **Cause**:
    - Deformed *cystic fibrosis trans-membrane conductance regulator (CFTR) gene* → abnormal protein → makes the **membrane impermeable to Cl⁻**
    - Cells lining the respiratory airways cannot absorb NaCl (salt) properly, → **salt accumulation→ leads to thick, excess mucus**
- **Treatment**:
    - **physical therapy** to get rid of the airways excess mucus
    - **antibiotics** to combat respiratory infections
    - Supplemental **pancreatic enzymes**

Cell to cell adhesions
Cells are held together by **(Fig. 31)**:
(a) tight junctions: form impermeable barrier

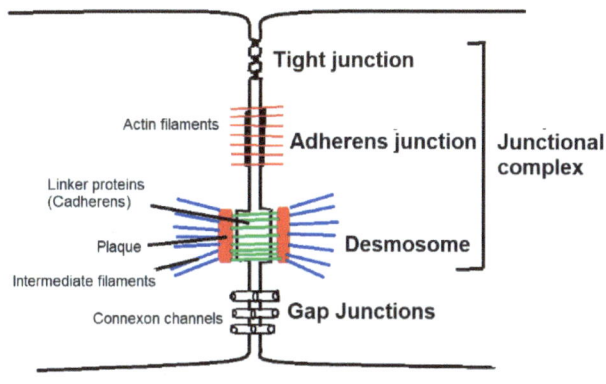

Figure 31: Gap junctions & Junctional complex

(b) Gap junctions allow materials to pass from cell to cell

- **2 connexons** (2 hollowed channels) join → form a hollow tube **(Fig. 32)**.
- **Function**: It permits passage of small, **water-soluble particles and ions**
- **Sites**: **cardiac** and **smooth** muscles, (for synchronized contraction).

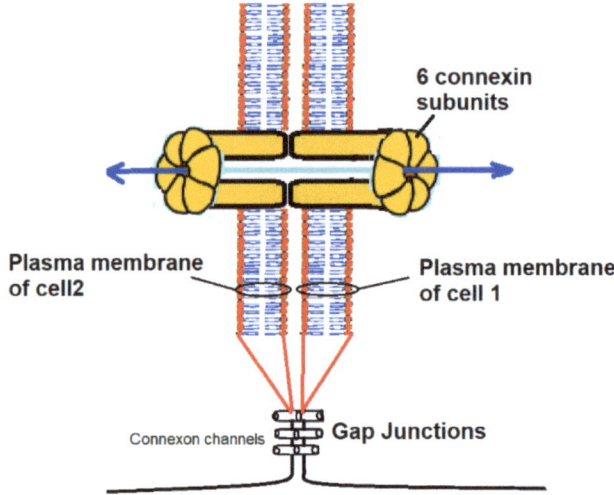

Figure 32: The structure of the gap junction (Connexons)

(c) Adhesion junctions (<u>desmosomes</u>) a button like structure that allow tissues to stretch.
- Desmosomes in the heart muscle cells prevent the cells from tearing apart during contraction.

Electric characters of the Cell membrane
   There is positive charge outside and negative charge inside ➡ membrane potential. Plasma membrane potential, action potential and graded potential are described in **chapter 5** (CNS & special senses).

III. Nucleus
- Is rounded or oval body, works as the control center of the cell.
- **Function**:
   - Provides the instructions for protein synthesis.
   - Transmits genetic information
- Have **3 regions**: nuclear envelope, nucleolus & chromatin.

1) Nuclear envelope:
- Double-membrane pierced by **pores**.

- **Pores** are lines by proteins, called a *nuclear pore complex*
- **Outer** membrane is continuous with the endoplasmic reticulum and contains ribosomes.
- The **inner** membrane is lined by the **nuclear Lamina**, a network of **lamins**

2) Nucleolus
- Is composed of **ribosomal RNA** and **proteins**.
- Is the site of ribosome subunit manufacture.
- Present around the DNA that codes for ribosomal RNA (rRNA) → combine with **proteins** → form the 2 types of ribosomal subunits.

3) Chromatin
- Granular, threadlike **DNA** + **histone proteins** → form **nucleosomes**.
- DNA forms the **genes**.
  - **Gene** = a segment of a DNA that carries instructions for creating one polypeptide chain.
  - Humans have about **20,000 genes** (form 2% of DNA).

nucleosomes:
- are the fundamental **units of chromatin**
- consist of **8 histone proteins**
- The **DNA** winds twice around each nucleosome and continues on to the next cluster via **linker DNA segments**
- **Active chromatin segments** are extended chromatin & cannot be seen under the light microscope.
- The **inactive condensed** chromatin segments are darkly stained and could be seen by light microscope.

Chromosomes
- Are short, bar like bodies formed in preparation of cell division.
- The chromatin threads coil and condense greatly to form chromosomes.

The Cell Cycle
- Consists of interphase & mitotic phase **(Fig. 33)**.

Interphase:
- the cell grows and carries its metabolic activities
- has **3 sub phases** G1, S & G2

G1 (gap 1 subphase):
- The cell can synthesize proteins and can grow.
- This is the most variable phase in length.
- Cells that permanently stop dividing are in the **G0 phase**.
- At its end, the centrioles start to replicate.

S (Synthetic):
- where **DNA replicate**

G2 (gap 2 subphase):
- This is usually a brief phase.
- Enzymes and proteins needed for division are synthesized.
- Centriole replication (begun in G1) is completed.
- G2/M checkpoint ensures that DNA is replicated.

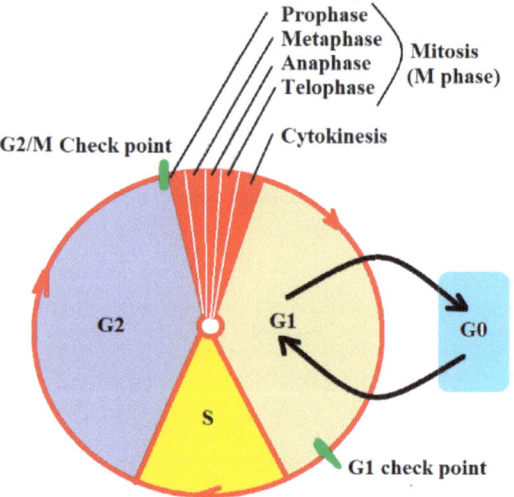

Figure 33: Cell cycle

DNA replication
  - DNA replication occurs during the **S phase**

Sequence of events:
- **Uncoiling**: Enzymes unwind the DNA molecule.
- **Separation**: The two DNA strands separate at a point known as the **replication fork**.
- **Assembly**: The 2 strands act as templates → the enzyme **DNA polymerase** puts complementary nucleotides along the template strands, forming 2 new (daughter) strands.
- **Restoration**: **Ligase** enzymes splice short segments of DNA together → restoring the **double helix** structure.

- Cells that lose their ability to divide are repaired with scar tissue (fibrous tissue)
  - nervous tissue
  - skeletal muscle
  - Heart muscle.

38

- **M (Mitotic) phase** of the cell cycle, have 2 events: mitosis and cytokinesis

Mitosis
- Normal body cell division
- It lasts about an hour or less.
- It has **4 phases**: **pro**phase, **meta**phase, **ana**phase & **telo**phase **(Fig. 34)**
- **Prophase**
    - Chromatin condenses → to form **chromosomes** (each formed of 2 **chromatids**, attached at **centromere**
    - Nucleoli disappear
    - Formation of **mitotic spindle** (microtubules).
    - Centrosomes separate
    - Nuclear envelope disappears
    - Chromosomes go to the equator of the cell

- **Metaphase**
    - The 2 **centrosomes** → pass to the 2 poles of the cell
    - Chromosomes cluster at the middle of the cell.
    - Enzymes separate the 2 chromatids from each other.
- **Anaphase**
    - Microtubules shorten to pull the chromosomes towards the 2 poles of the cell.
- **Telophase**
    - Chromosomes uncoil → give chromatin network.
    - Spindle disappears.
    - Formation of new nuclear envelope.

Cytokinesis
= the division of the cytoplasm.
- Actin filaments draw the plasma membrane inward → **forming** contractile ring with a **cleavage furrow** at the center of the cell.
- The furrow deepens → it divides the cytoplasm into 2 parts→ giving **2 daughter cells** (which are smaller)

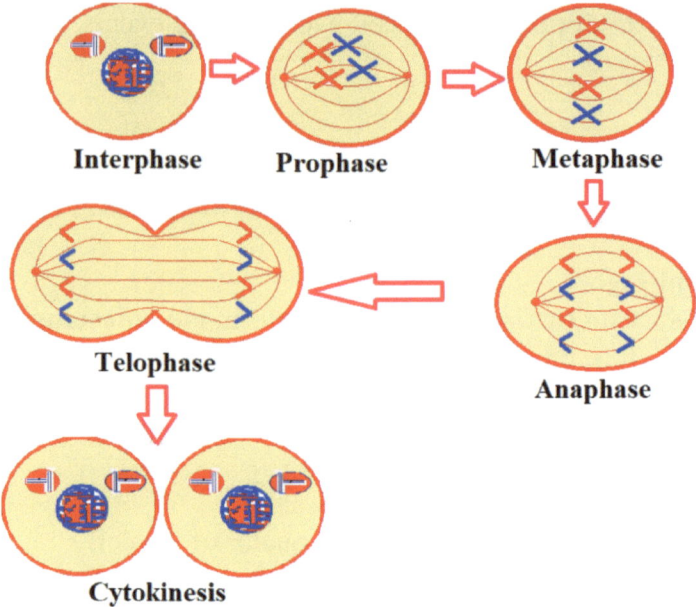

Figure 34: Cell division (mitosis)

<u>Meiosis</u> = reduction division
- Produces sex cells (ova and sperms) with only **half the number of genes** found in body cells.

Protein synthesis
- Protein is synthesized from **DNA genes**, helped by **RNA**

<u>Ganes</u>
- Each 3 bases (called **triplet)** code for a particular **amino acid**
  - AAA code for phenylalanine
  - CCT code for glycine
- The coding regions are called **exons**.
- Exons are separated by **introns** (work as control elements)

<u>RNA</u>

3 forms of RNA:
- **Messenger RNA (mRNA)**
  - nucleotide resembling "half-DNA" molecule
  - Carries the code from the nuclear chromatin to the cytoplasm.
- **Ribosomal RNA (rRNA)**
  - Is formed in the **nucleolus**.
  - Consists of two **subunits**, one **large** and one **small**.
  - Is the site of protein synthesis.
- **Transfer RNA (tRNA)**

- small, L-shaped molecules
- It transfers amino acids to the ribosomes.
- In the ribosomes they decode mRNA's message to build the polypeptide.

Protein synthesis: includes 2 processes; transcription + translation
<u>**Transcription**</u>
= transferring information from **DNA** to complementary **mRNA (Fig. 35)**
It passes through **3 stages**:
- **Initiation**: **RNA polymerase** binds to the **promoter**, separates the two DNA strands, and initiates mRNA synthesis.
- **Elongation**: RNA polymerase elongates the mRNA, unwinding the DNA double helix in front and rewinding it behind.
- **Termination**: mRNA synthesis ends when the polymerase reaches a **termination signal** (special nucleotide sequence).

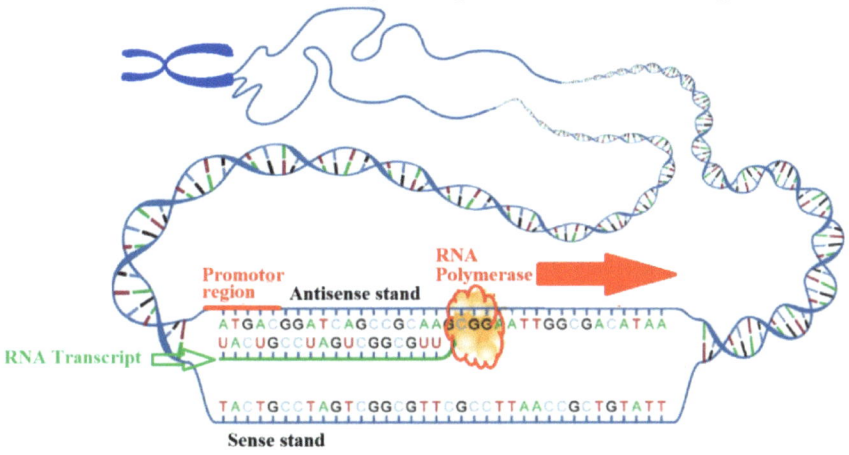

Figure 35: Transcription

<u>**Translation**</u>
Translate the **mRNA** into **protein** (amino acid sequence).
<u>Components of translation</u>
- **Genetic Code:**
    - Is the base sequence of a gene
- **codon:**
    - is the 3 base sequence on mRNA **(Fig. 36)**
- **tRNA**
    - tRNA is shaped like a handheld drill.
    - one end binds to an **amino acid**
    - the opposite end carries **anticodon**, which binds to the mRNA codon **(Fig. 36)**

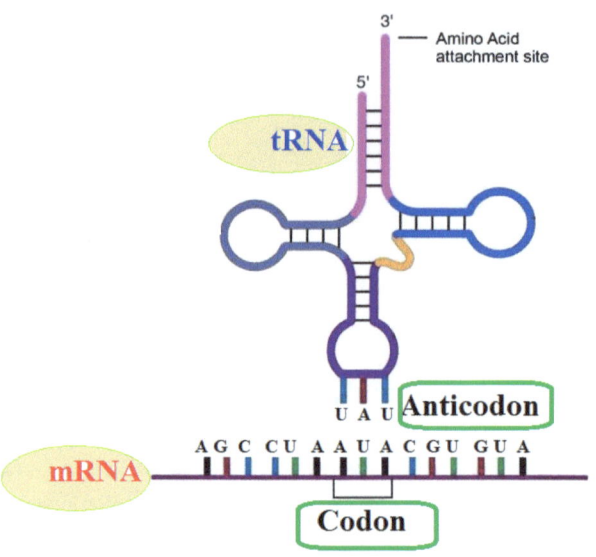

Figure 36: Codon in mRNA & anticodon in tRNA

Ribosome

- has one binding site for **mRNA** and three binding sites for **tRNA**: **(Fig. 37)**
    - **A (aminoacyl)** for an aminoacyl-tRNA
    - **P (peptidyl)** site for the tRNA holding the growing polypeptide chain
    - **E (exit)** site for an outgoing tRNA

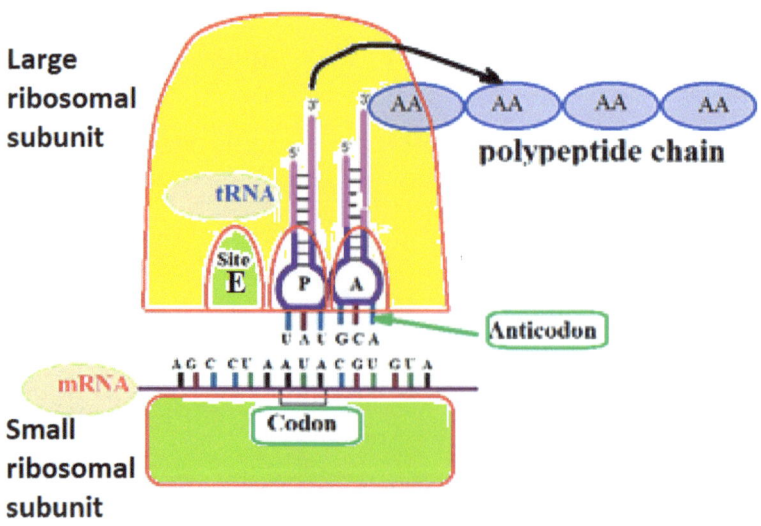

Figure 37: Formation of polypeptide chain

Sequence of Events in Translation
- **Initiation**: 4 components combine
  - A small ribosomal subunit
  - A large ribosomal subunit
  - tRNA carrying the amino acid
  - mRNA
- **Elongation**: Amino acids are added to the growing peptide chain in a repeating steps:
  - **Codon recognition**: the anticodon (of the tRNA) binds with the codon (of the complementary mRNA)
  - **Peptide bond formation**: The growing polypeptide bound to the tRNA at the **P site** → is transferred to the amino acid carried by the tRNA in the **A site** → new peptide bond is formed.
- **Translocation**: The entire ribosome translocate → shifting its position one codon along the mRNA.
- **Termination**: When a stop codon (UGA, UAA, or UAG) arrives at the A site, elongation ends.

DNA Finger printing
  = DNA identification technology
- The composition of DNA is unique to each individual (like fingerprints).
- Identical twins only share the same DNA.
- Samples are taken from Blood, hair, bone, tissue, nail clippings, saliva, etc.
- DNA is digested into fragments of differing sizes using **restriction enzymes**
- Gel **electrophoresis** separates the DNA (with negative charges) → DNA fragments separate according to size
- This technique identifies "**short tandem repeats (STRs)**"
  - STRs are segments of repeating nucleotides (for example, A-A-A-A or T-T-T-T).
  - Their exact location is unique to each individual.
- Each STR is tagged with **radioactive molecules** → **the** labeled gel is exposed to **X ray film**→ giving pattern similar to the "**bar code**," with alternating light and dark bands.

Section 4: Tissues, Organs & Systems

Tissues
- Are groups of cells with similar structure & function
- **4 types** of tissues:
(1) **Epithelial tissue**: covers surfaces & lines cavities
(2) **Connective tissue:** binds and supports body parts
(3) **Muscular tissue:** contracts
(4) **Nervous tissue:** responds to stimuli and communicates
  - "**4Cs**" mnemonic: *Cover-Connect-Contract-Communicate.*
  - Organs are usually composed of all the 4 types.

Epithelial tissue
- Function:
  - Covering & protection
  - exchanging materials, secretion, absorption
- organized into two types of structures:
  - **epithelial** sheets
  - **Secretory** glands

Epithelial sheets (Fig. 38)
- **Simple**: one layer of cells
  - Simple squamous (flat cells): as capillaries, alveoli
  - Simple cuboidal: as glands
  - Simple columnar (tall cells)
- **Stratified**: several layers of cells, named according to the surface cells
  - Stratified squamous: as skin
  - Stratified cuboidal: as ducts of glands
  - **Pseudostratified** columnar: long + short cells, all the cells reach the basement membrane: as respiratory epithelium.
- **Transitional**: surface layer is dome-shaped: as urinary tract
  - appear in 2 forms: contracted or flat (extended)

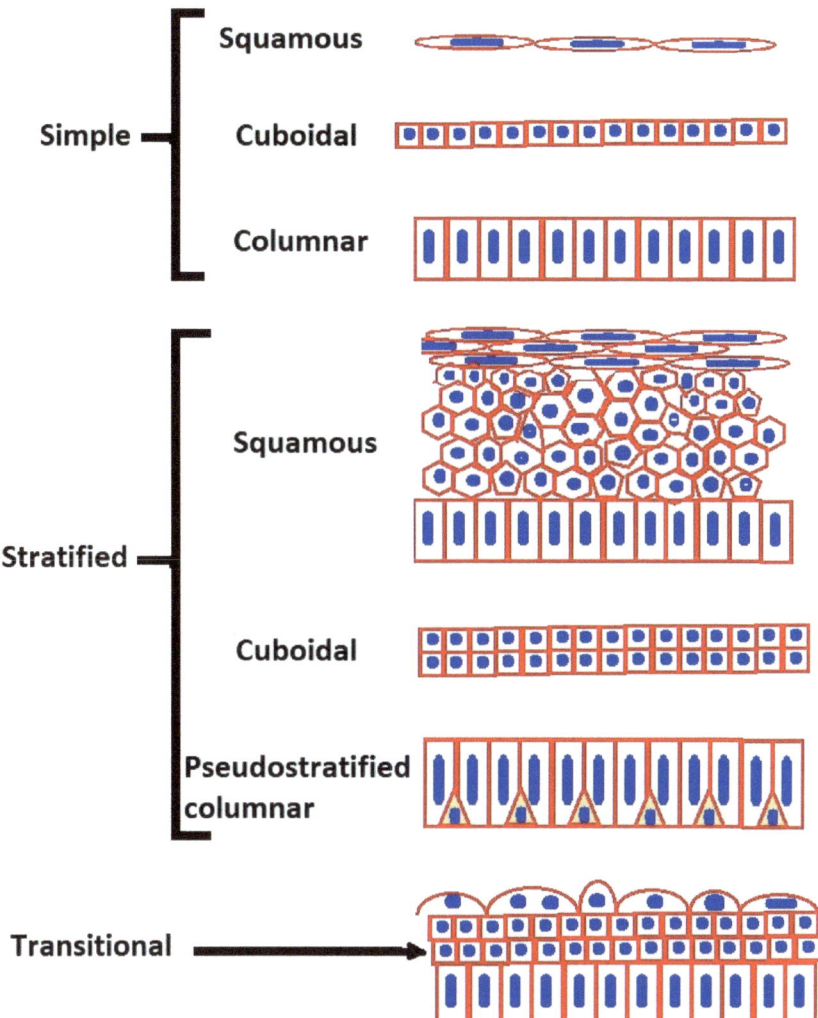

Figure 38: Types of epithelium

<u>**Glands**</u>
- formed of epithelial tissue specialized for secretion.

<u>**Classification**</u>
- **Endocrine**: have no duct, secrete hormones into blood
- **Exocrine**: have ducts, secrete to the surface or cavities
  - ❏ Examples: sweat glands, glands of GIT
  - ❏ Types: **(Fig. 39)**
    - – **Simple** (one duct + one secretory part): tubular, alveolar, coiled
    - – **Branched** (one duct + several secretory parts): tubular, alveolar

— **Compound** (duct is branched + several secretory parts): tubular, alveolar

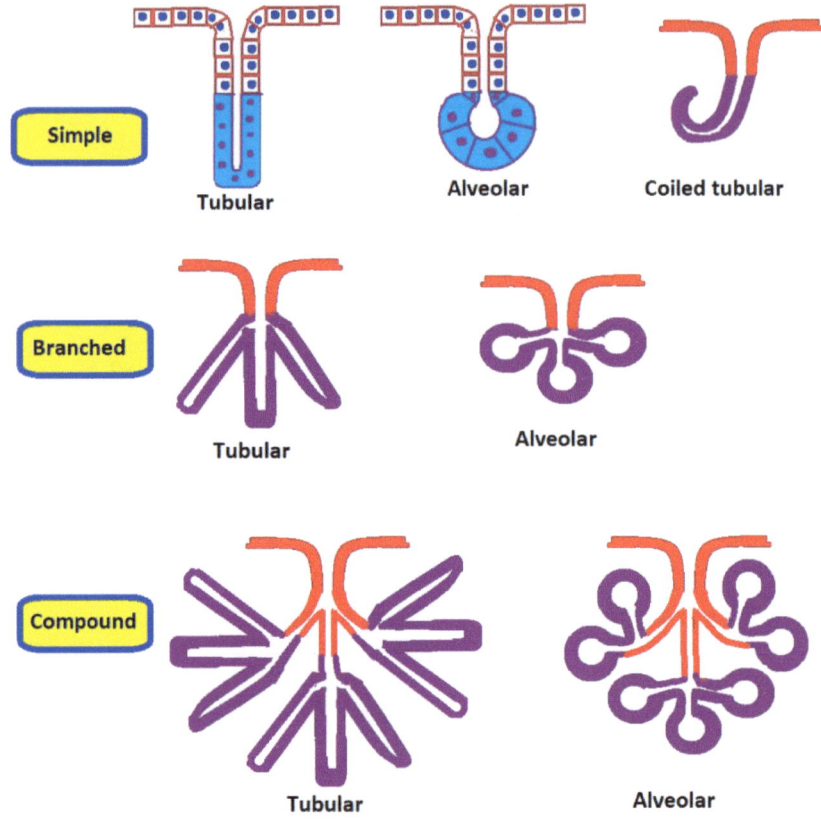

Figure 39: Types of glands

<u>**Clinical note**</u>
- In long-term smokers, the **pseudostratified ciliated columnar** epithelium in the bronchi → is gradually converted to **stratified squamous epithelium**.

Connective tissue (CT)

Function:
- binds structures together
- supports and protects
- fills spaces
- stores fat

Structure:
- few **cells** (fibroblasts)

+ Extracellular **matrix** (*organic ground substance* + *fibers*).
- 3 types of **fibers**:
  - **Collagen:** gives the fibers flexibility and strength.
  - **Elastic:** contain *elastin,* which is elastic.
  - **Reticular:** delicate, thin, highly branched, supporting networks.

Classification of Connective tissue
1. Loose CT
   - Areolar
   - Adipose
2. Dense CT
   - Dense regular
   - Dense irregular
   - Yellow elastic
3. Reticular CT
4. Cartilage
5. Bone
6. Blood

1. Loose CT (Fig. 40)
Loose areolar CT
- Location: Between tissues and organs
- Function: Binds tissues and organs together
- Structure: fibroblasts + collagen & elastic fs + jelly like ground substance

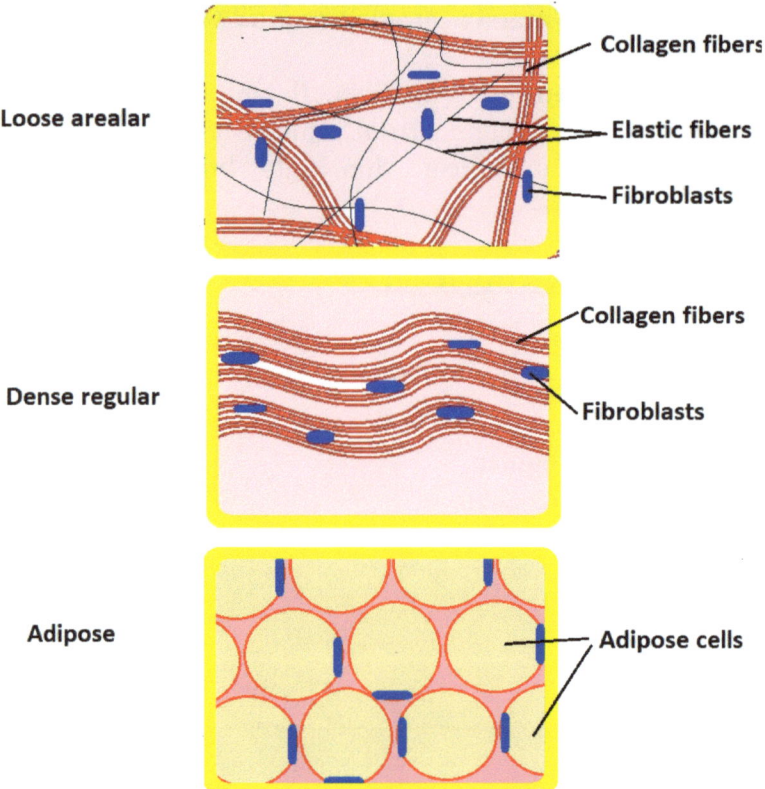

Figure 40: Connective tissue proper

Adipose tissue
- Have fat cells (adipocytes) + limited extracellular matrix.

2. Dense CT
Dense regular
- Contains parallel collagen bundles
- Fibroblasts between the bundles
- found in tendons, ligaments and aponeuroses

Dense irregular
- Collagen fires run in different directions
- found in the *dermis* of the skin and in joint capsules

Elastic CT
- Contains elastic fibers, capable of stretching
- found in
  - walls of the largest arteries

       –   vocal cords

3. Reticular CT:
- Contains **reticular cells**, and reticular fibers
- When it contains WBCs (lymphocytes) it is called **lymphatic tissue**

4. Cartilage
- The cells are called *chondrocytes*
  - lie in **lacunae** (small chambers)
  - Are formed from *chondroblasts, which* help cartilage to grow
- Cells are separated by **matrix** (solid & flexible)
- Cartilages have no blood supply, therefore heals very slowly.
- 3 types of cartilages according to the type of fibers in the matrix: hyaline, elastic and fibrous **(Fig. 41)**

1) Hyaline cartilage
- Is strong, durable & flexible.
- The matrix contains very fine **collagen fibers**
- Is **found in** the nose, ends of the long bones, ribs, trachea, fetal skeleton

2) Elastic cartilage
- Its matrix contains many elastic fibers, in addition to collagen fibers.
- It is more flexible than hyaline cartilage.
- Found in external ear, and epiglottis

3) Fibrocartilage
- Its matrix contains strong collagen fibers
- Its function is to absorbs shock, withstand tension and pressure
- Found in the intervertebral disc and knee menisci

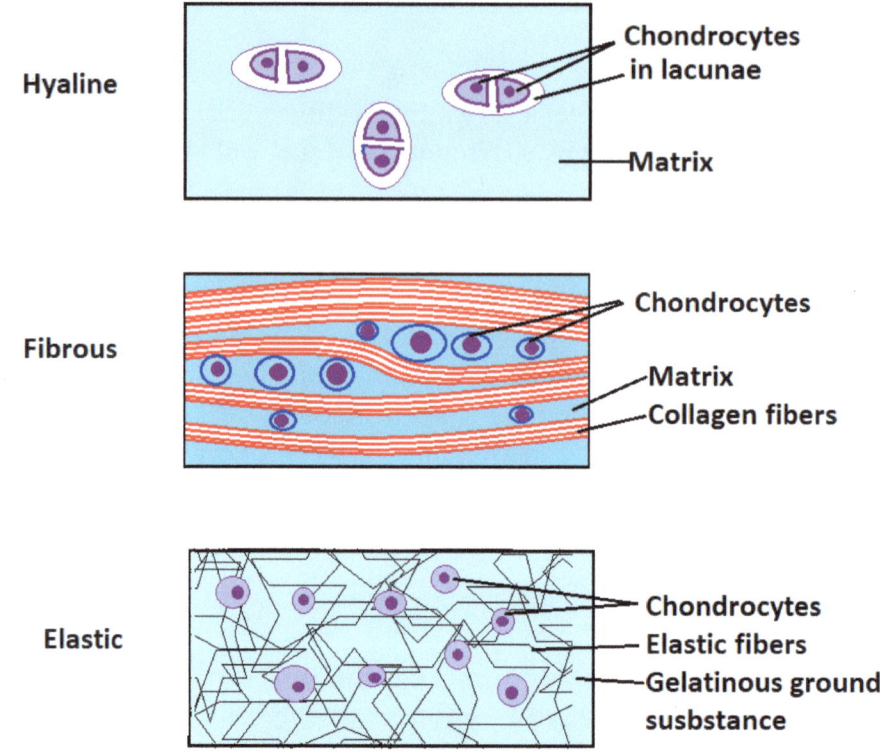

Figure 41: Types of cartilages

<u>Growth of cartilage</u>:
- **appositional growth**: deposit matrix on the surface from the perichondrium
- **interstitial growth**: expanding from inside

5. Bones
<u>Functions</u>
- **Support** the body
- **Protect** soft structures
- **Attachment** of skeletal muscles
- **Mineral storage**: calcium, Phosphate
- **Blood formation**: in red marrow
- **Storage of fat**: in yellow marrow
- **Hormone** production: **osteocalcin** (regulates insulin secretion).

<u>Classification of bones</u>
- **According to shape:**
  - **Long** bones: bones of the limbs, have 2 ends + shaft

50

- **Short** bones: bones of wrist & ankle
- **Flat** bones: bones of the skull, ribs, sternum, scapula
- **Irregular** bones: vertebrae, hip bone
- **According to position:**
  - **Axial** skeleton: vertebrae, skull, ribs
  - **Appendicular**: limbs, girdles
- **According to structure: (Fig. 42)**
  - **Compact**: dense bone, e.g. shaft of long bone, arranged in concentric layers of units called **osteons (Haversian system) (Fig. 43)**
  - **Spongy**: trabecular, filled with red or yellow marrow

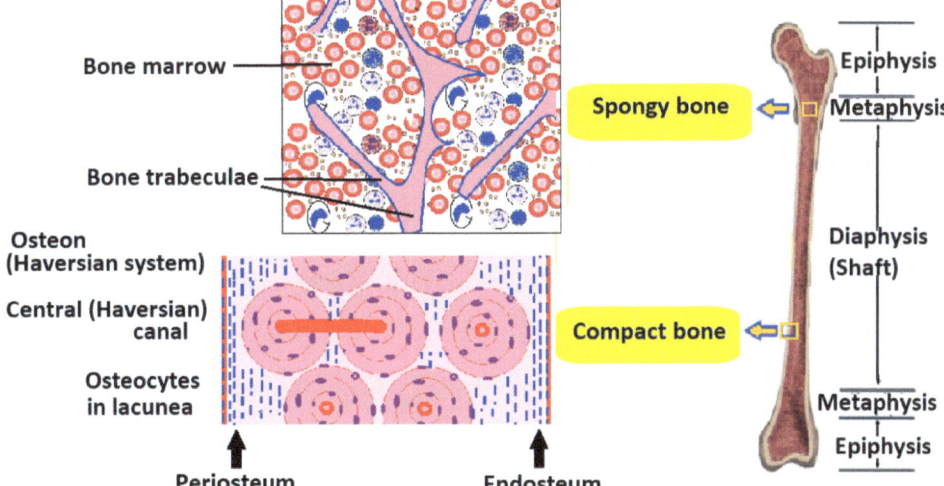

Figure 42: Compact and spongy bones

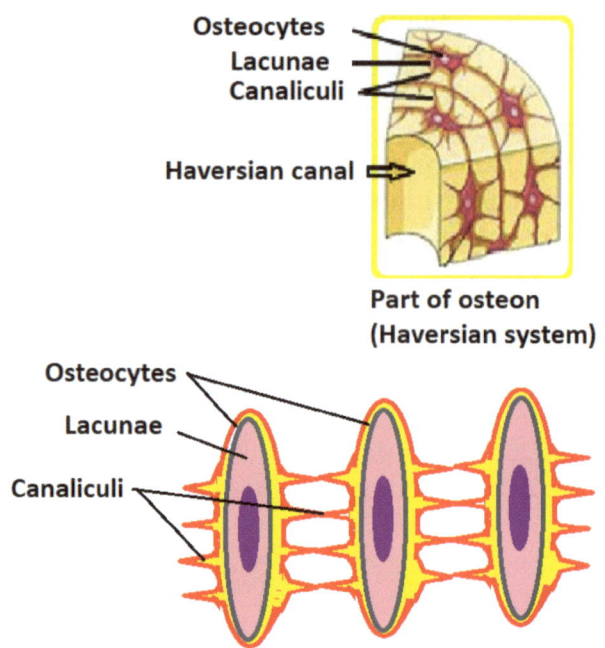

Osteocytes
Lacunae
Canaliculi

Haversian canal ⇨

Part of osteon
(Haversian system)

Osteocytes

Lacunae

Canaliculi

Figure 43: Structure of compact bone

Structure of long bone (Fig. 44)

- Shaft = **diaphysis**: contains compact bone, then spongy bone, surrounding marrow cavity
- 2 ends = **epiphysis**: compact & spongy bones, covered with hyaline cartilage
- Epiphyseal **line**: between epiphysis & diaphysis, is a remnant of the epiphyseal plate (growth plate)
- **Periosteum**: contains osteoblasts & osteoclasts
- **Endosteum**: lines the marrow cavity

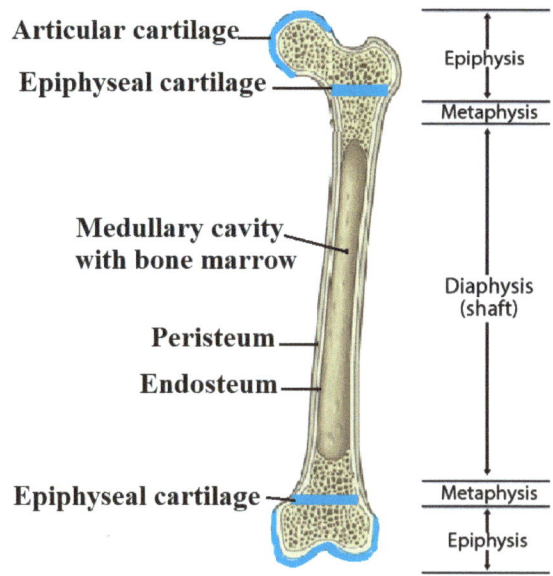

Figure 44: Structure of long bone

Cells of bone tissue (Fig. 45)

   a) **osteogenic** cells = active stem cells → divide & give osteoblasts
   b) **osteoblasts**: → secrete bone matrix (osteoid) & give osteocytes
   c) **osteocytes**: present inside lacunae and have canaliculi, maintain bone matrix
   d) **osteoclasts**: → have ruffled border, give bone resorption

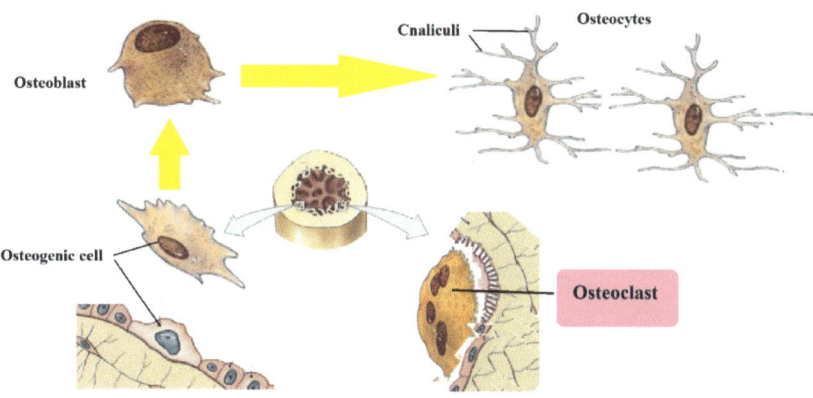

Figure 45: Cells of bone tissue

Chemical composition of bone

   • **Organic**: cells + osteoid (ground substance + collagen)
   • **Inorganic** (65%): hydroxyapatite (calcium phosphate)

Bone ossification

- **Endochondral ossification**: occur in long bones, by replacing hyaline cartilage **(Fig. 46)**
  - ❑ In the **diaphysis**: → forms bone collar + primary ossification center
  - ❑ Medullary cavity develops & primary ossification center enlarges
  - ❑ In **epiphysis** → secondary ossification center develops
  - ❑ **Hyaline cartilage** remains in
    - – Epiphyseal plate: → allows growth of length
    - – Articular cartilage: → to form joints
- **Intramembranous ossification**: bone replaces fibrous membrane

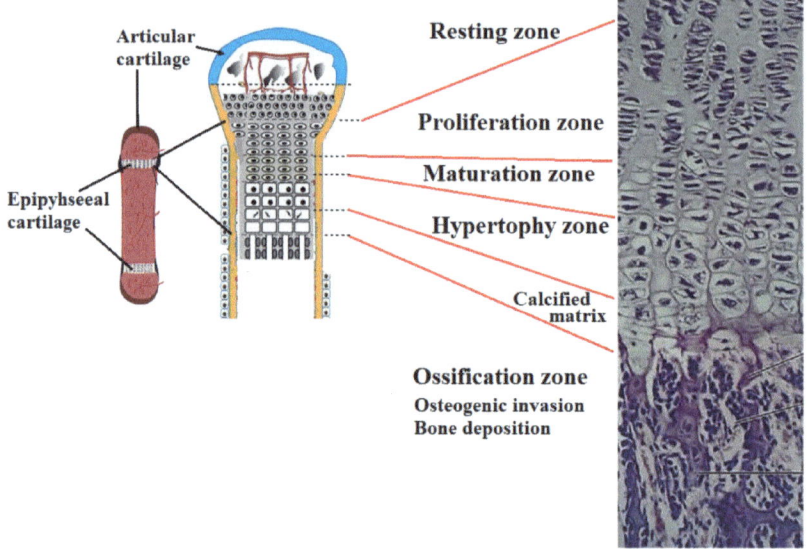

Figure 46: Endochondral ossification

Repair of bone: passes through the following stages
1) **Hematoma** formation →
2) **Fibrocartilaginous callus** formation →
3) **Bony callus** formation →
4) **Bone remodeling**: resorption of bone excess

Bone disorders

- **Osteomalacia**: poorly mineralized, soft, weak bones
  - – treated with calcium & vitamin D
- **Rickets**: the same in children
  - – gives bowed legs
- **Osteoporosis**: bone resorption more than bone deposition
  - – Occur in menopause women

- **Paget's disease**: excessive abnormal bone resorption and deposition
    - gives deformity

6. Blood

- Blood is a connective tissue composed of **formed elements (cells)** suspended in a **liquid matrix** called **plasma**.
- **3 formed elements**: **(Fig. 47)**
    1. red blood cells (**RBCs/ erythrocytes**) → carry oxygen
    2. white blood cells (**WBCs/ leukocytes**) → fight infection
    3. platelets (**thrombocytes**),
        - are fragments of **megakaryocytes**
        - function: blood clotting.

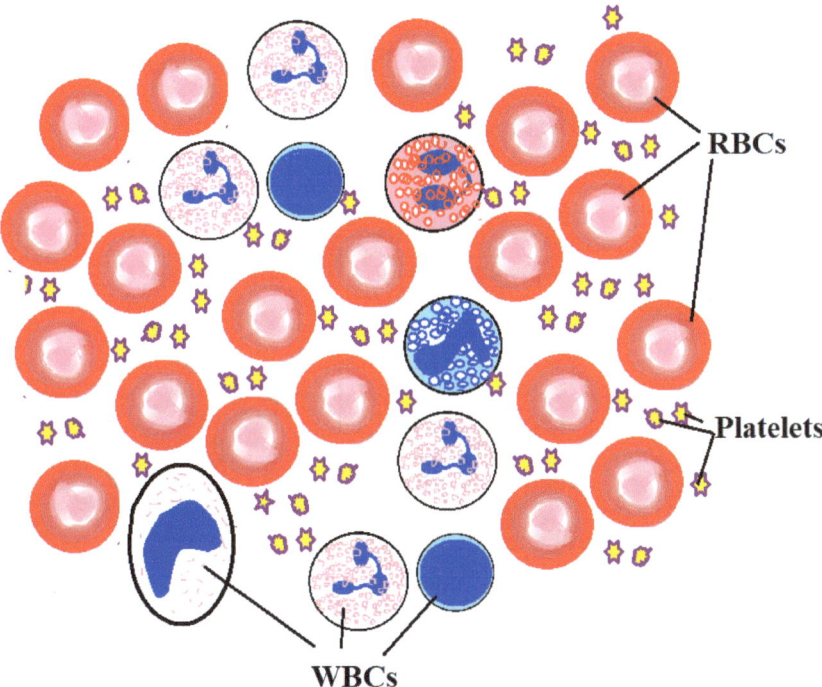

Figure 47: Blood picture

Muscle tissue

Specialized for contraction → generating force
3 types (Fig. 48)

- **Skeletal** muscle

- Moves the skeleton
- **Cardiac** muscle
  - Pumps blood out of the heart
- **Smooth** muscle
  - controls hollow tubes and organs
  - Example: digestive tract

by light microscope
- **Striated:** have alternating dark and light bands (example: skeletal and cardiac muscles)
- **Non-striated** (smooth muscle)

Innervation
- **voluntary** (skeletal muscle) supplied by somatic nerves
- **involuntary** (cardiac and smooth muscles), autonomic nerves

Skeletal muscle (Fig. 48)
- Shortens → to move the skeleton
- Under voluntary control
- They are formed by fusion of several cells → giving a long fiber with multiple nuclei under the plasma membrane (subsarcolemmal nuclei).
- The fibers have alternating light and dark bands (due to alternating actin and myosin filaments) → give them a *striated* appearance.

Levels of organization: arranged from large to small
- **Muscle** → consists of
- **Muscle fibers:** extend along the entire length of the muscle →
- **Myofibrils:** extend along the entire length of the muscle →
- **Myofilaments** (contractile elements):
  - **thick filaments**: protein **myosin**
  - **thin filaments**: protein **actin**
- **Electron Microscope:** shows alternating **dark bands** (the **A** bands) and **light bands** (the **I** bands)

Cardiac muscle (Fig. 48)
- The fibers branch and unite with each other
- Fibers have central nucleus

- Characterized by the **intercalated discs (desmosomes + gap junctions)** between adjacent cells → permit rapid spread of contractile stimuli
- it has striations
- the contraction is *involuntary*
- It pumps blood out of the heart

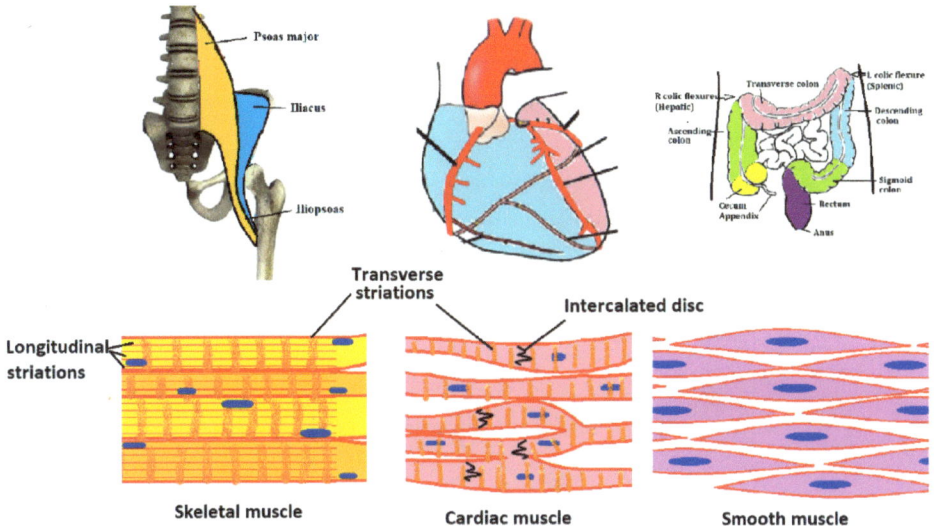

Figure 48: Types of muscles

Smooth muscle (Fig. 48)

- Cells are **spindle-shaped**, thick at the middle
- with central oval nucleus
- The arrangement of actin and myosin does not give striations.
- Sites:
  - present in the walls of the hollow organs as blood vessels, digestive tube, urinary bladder, uterus

Skeletal muscle	Cardiac muscle	Smooth muscle
striated, cylindrical, Multinucleated fibers	striated, cylindrical, branched fibers, with one or two nuclei	spindle-shaped fibers, with single nucleus
Location: attached to skeleton or skin	**Location**: heart wall	**Location**: walls of hollow organs (e.g., stomach, intestines, urinary bladder, uterus, blood vessels)
NS: somatic	**NS:** autonomic	**NS:** autonomic
Control: voluntary	**Control**: involuntary	**Control**: involuntary

Nervous tissue

- **Nervous tissue**
  - Found in brain, spinal cord, nerves and special sense organs.
  - Contain nerve cells (**neurons**) + **neuroglia** cells.

Neurons (= nerve cells) (Fig. 49)

- Initiate and transmit electrical impulses
- Relay information from one part of the body to another.
- It has 3 parts:

  (1) **Dendrites** receives impulses

  (2) **Cell body** contains the nucleus and the cytoplasm

  (3) **Axon** conducts impulses. It forms:
  - *tracts* in the brain & spinal cord
  - **nerves** in the peripheral nervous system.

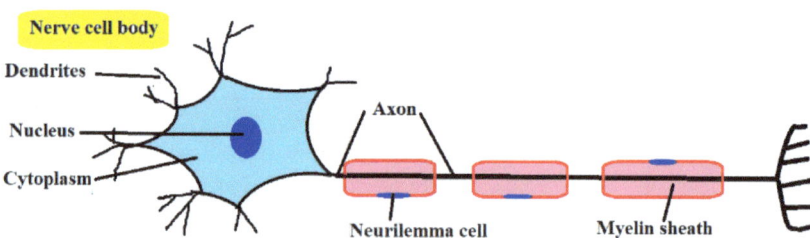

Figure 49: Nerve cell

Neuroglia (Glial) cells (Fig. 50)

1) Astrocytes

Are the most abundant glial cells.

Function:

    1. Act as the main "**glue**" of the CNS

    2. Guides neurons to their final destination **during fetal development.**

    3. Establish the **blood–brain barrier**

    4. Transfer **nutrients** from the blood

    5. Repair brain injuries by forming neural scars.

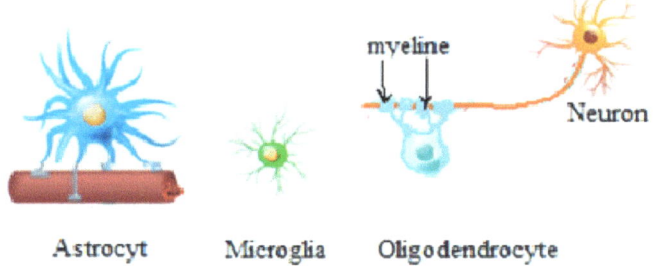

myeline

Neuron

Astrocyt   Microglia   Oligodendrocyte

Figure 50: Neuroglia cells

2) Microglia
- Immune cells of the CNS.
- Function: Phagocytosis and release of destructive chemicals, as in stroke, Alzheimer's disease, multiple sclerosis

3) Oligodendrocytes
- Formation of **myelin sheaths** around axons in the CNS.
- This role is done by Schwann cells in PNS

4) Ependymal cells
- **Line the cavities** of the brain and spinal cord
- Form barrier between CSF and tissue fluid of the CNS

Organs
- Consist of two or more types of primary tissues that function together to perform certain functions
- Example: **Stomach**
  - Is lined with **epithelial tissue**
  - Its wall contains smooth **muscle, glands & nervous** tissue
  - **Connective tissue** binds all the above tissues together

Body systems
- **Systems** are groups of organs that perform related functions.
- **For example**, the **digestive system** consists of the mouth, pharynx (throat), esophagus, stomach, small intestine, large intestine, salivary glands, exocrine pancreas, liver, and gallbladder.
- Human body has **11 systems** that could be classified into 4 categories: **(Fig. 51)**
  - **Support, Movement, and Protection**
    1. Integumentary system: skin + glands
    2. Skeletal system: axial & appendicular

   3. Muscular system: skeletal, cardiac & smooth
- **Integration and Coordination**
  1. Nervous system
  2. Endocrine system
- **Maintenance of the Body**
  1. Cardiovascular system
  2. Lymphatic system
  3. Respiratory system
  4. Digestive system
  5. Urinary system
- **Reproduction &Development**
  - Male & female reproductive systems

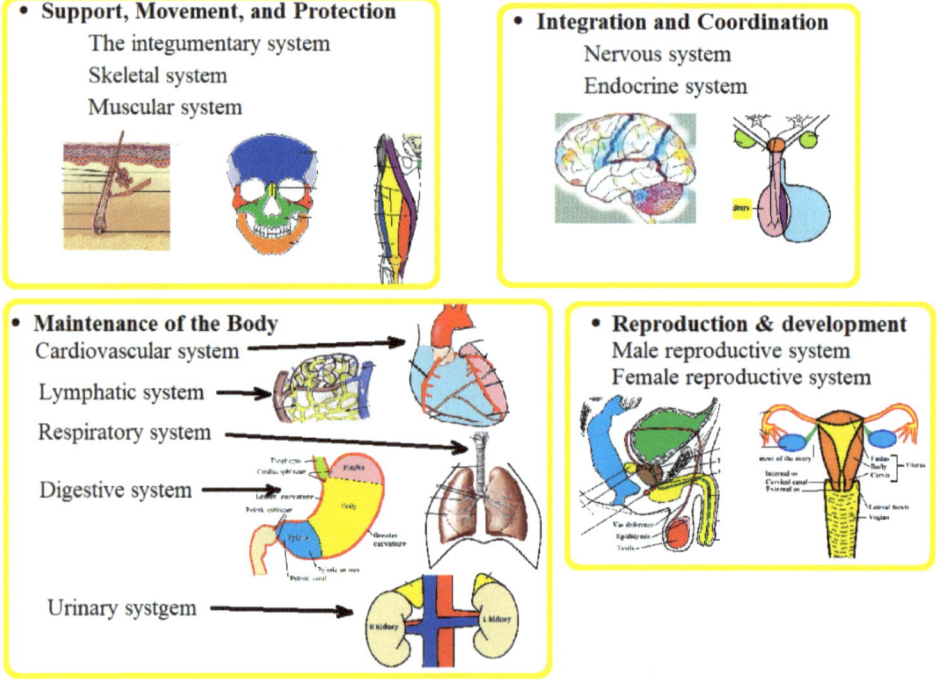

Figure 51: Organ/ system organization

Section 5: Introduction to Anatomy

- **Anatomy** is the study of the structure of the body, in order to understand the function.
- Its basics include
  - Anatomical position
  - Terms of position
  - Anatomical planes
  - Anatomical regions
  - Anatomical quadrants

<u>**Anatomical position**</u>
- The **body stands upright with the** face looking forward, **feet together, arms by the sides, palms facing forward** and the **thumbs** pointing away from the body **(Fig. 52)**
- It is the position of the body for describing the structure
- it resembles "standing at attention"
- Other positions
  - **Prone position**: the body is lying face down
  - **Supine position**: the body is lying face up

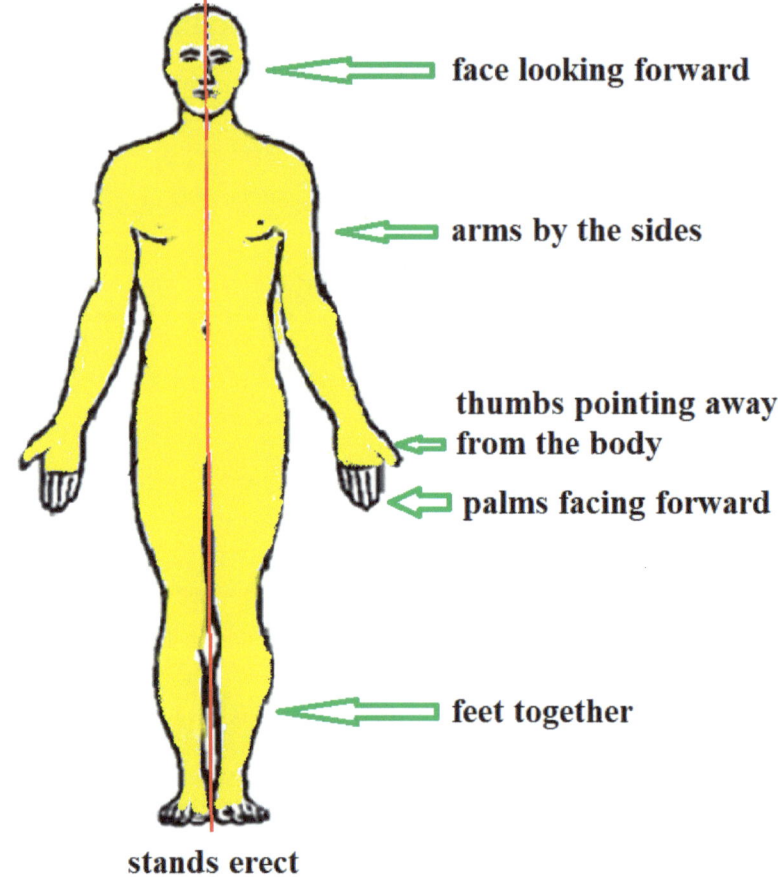

face looking forward

arms by the sides

thumbs pointing away from the body

palms facing forward

feet together

stands erect

Figure 52: Anatomical position

<u>**Terms of position**</u>
Describes the position of one part in relation to another part **(Fig. 53)**
- **Superior** (cranial): towards the head
- **Inferior** (caudal): away from the head
    - Example: the lung is superior to the liver, the liver lies inferior to the lung

- **Anterior** (ventral): near the front of the body
- **Posterior** (dorsal): near the back of the body
    - Example: the heart is anterior to the spine, the spine lies posterior to the heart

- **Medial**: near the midline
- **Lateral**: away from the midline
- **Intermediate**: between medial & lateral

- Example: the ulna is medial to the radius and the radius is lateral to the ulna

- **Proximal**: near the trunk
- **Distal**: away from the trunk
  - Example: the arm is proximal to the forearm

- **Superficial** (external): towards the surface of the body
- **Deep** (internal): away from the surface of the body
  - Example: the ribs lie deep to the skin

- **Midline**: imaginary vertical line that divides the body into right and left equal halves

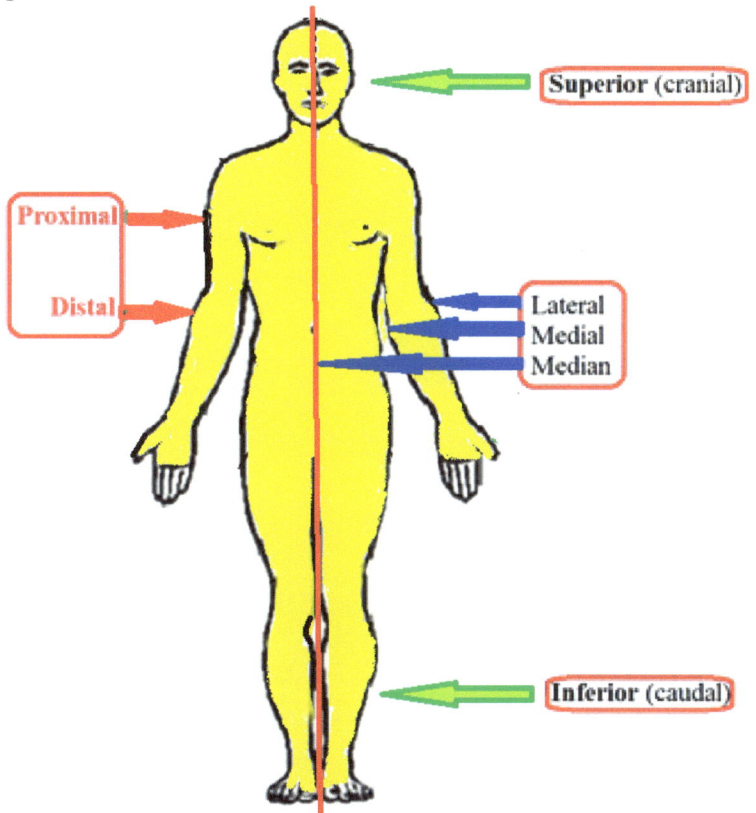

Figure 53: Terms of position

Anatomical planes: (Fig. 54)
- **Sagittal plane**: vertical plane that divides the body into right & left parts

- **Median sagittal** (midsagittal) plane: is a sagittal plane that passes through the midline and divides the body into right & left equal halves
- **Parasagittal** plane: sagittal plane that passes to the side of the midline
- **Coronal** (frontal) plane: vertical plane that divides the body into anterior & posterior parts
- **Transverse** plane = horizontal plane = cross-section: divides the body into superior & inferior parts

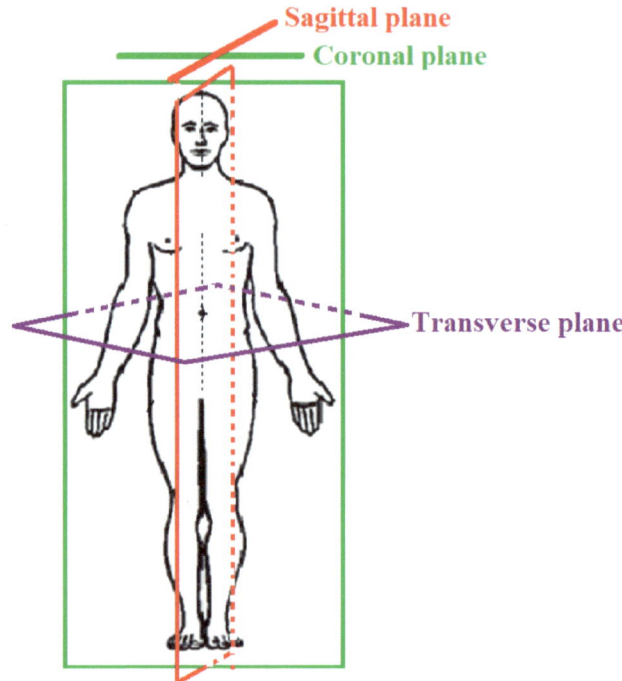

Figure 54: Anatomical planes

Anatomical regions

- Are 9 regions **(Fig. 55)**, formed by 4 lines (or planes)
  - 2 vertical lines: midclavicular lines (Rt & Lt)
  - 2 horizontal lines
    - Subcostal line: just inferior to the ribs
    - Intertubercular line: between the tubercles of iliac crest
- The **right and left iliac regions** lie lateral to the **hypogastric** region.
- The right and left **lumbar regions** lie lateral to the **umbilical** region.
- The right and left **hypochondriac regions** lie lateral to the **epigastric** region, deep to the ribs.

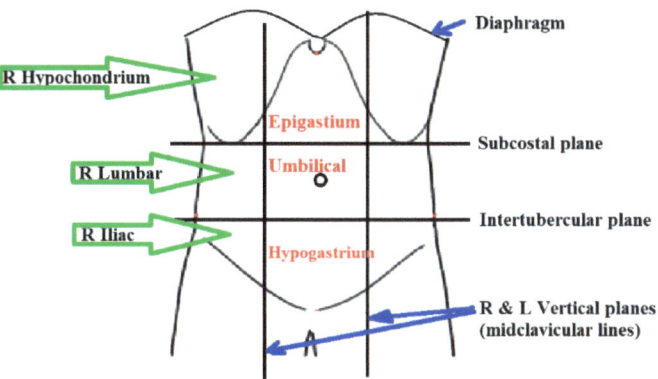

Figure 55: Anatomical regions

Anatomical quadrants

- Produced by 2 lines passing through the umbilicus: **(Fig. 56)**
  - one median vertical line
  - one horizontal line
1) right upper quadrant (RUQ)
2) left upper quadrant (LUQ)
3) right lower quadrant (RLQ)
4) left lower quadrant (LLQ)

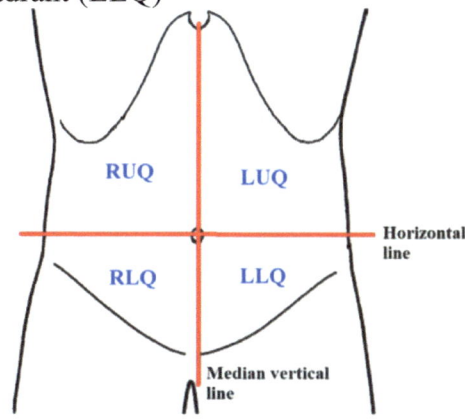

Figure 56: Anatomical quadrants

Body cavities & membranes (Fig. 57)
Posterior (Dorsal) Body Cavity

- Is subdivided into
  - (1) **Cranial cavity**, contains the brain
  - (2) **Vertebral canal**, contains the spinal cord
- Lined by 3 membranes (meninges)
  - Dura mater
  - Arachnoid mater

o Pia mater

Anterior (Ventral) Body Cavity

Is subdivided into
- superior thoracic cavity
- inferior abdominopelvic cavity

Lined by **serous membranes**
- In the thorax:
  - o **Pericardium**: around the heart
  - o **Pleura**: around the lungs
- In the abdomen & pelvis: **peritoneum**
- The serous membranes are like a balloon, pushed by the organs, to have 2 layers:
  - o **Visceral layer**: around the organ
  - o **Parietal layer**: lining the body wall
  - o There is **serous fluid** between the 2 layers, to lubricate the movement

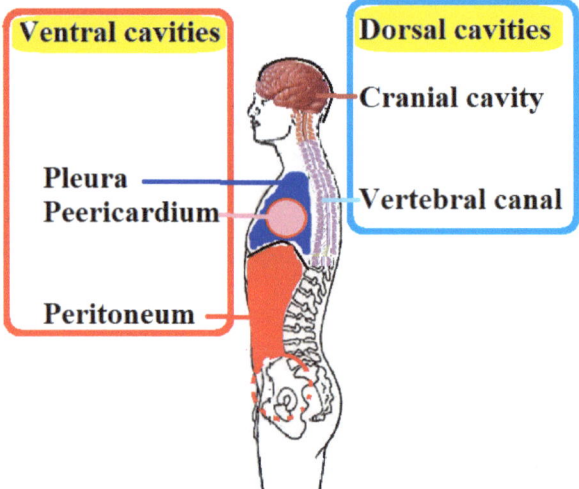

Figure 57: Body cavities

Clinical correlation

Inflammation (itis) of the lining membranes
- Anterior (Ventral) Body Cavity
  Serositis: inflammation of the serous membranes
  - – **Pericarditis**
  - – **Pleurisy**
  - – **Peritonitis**
- Posterior (Dorsal) Body Cavity
  - – **Meningitis**

Medical Imaging

- Techniques which create images of the body
- **X-ray** (radiography): bones appear radiopaque (white), while hollow structures as lung appear radio translucent (black)
  - **Mammography**: uses low dose x-ray
  - **Angiography**: uses contrast x-ray to create image of blood vessels
  - Computed Tomography (**CT**) **Scans**: use x-ray beam around the body → computer creates cross sectional view
- Magnetic Resonance Imaging (**MRI**): uses high energy magnetic field → resonates the hydrogen protons → a pulse of radio wave reads the pattern
- **Ultrasound** Imaging: high frequency sound waves → are reflected off the body tissues → detected by the same instrument
  - **Doppler** ultrasound: observe blood flow in vessels
- Positron Emission Tomography (**PET**) **Scans:** a substance is injected into the body → emits positrons (positively charged) that collide with electrons (negatively charged), → emit **gamma rays** → detected by **gamma camera**

Section 6: Introduction to Physiology

Physiology
- Is the study of the body **functions**
- The functions of all the systems contribute to the **homeostasis**

Homeostasis:
- **Definition**: It is the maintenance of a stable internal environment that surround the cells (extracellular fluid, ECF)
- It is the main goal of Physiology
- Cells exchange oxygen and nutrients with **tissue fluid** → then with **blood** → to maintain the internal environment

Contributions of Body Systems to Homeostasis
- Circulatory system
  - Carries materials from one part of the body to another
- Digestive system
  - Breaks down dietary **food** into smaller molecules that can be absorbed & distributed to body cells
  - Transfers **water** and **electrolytes** from external environment to internal environment
  - Eliminates undigested food **residues** to external environment in the feces
- Respiratory system
  - Gets O_2 and eliminates CO_2
  - maintenance of the **pH** of internal environment
- Urinary system
  - Removes excess water, salt, acid, and other electrolytes
- Skeletal system
  - Provides support and protection for soft tissues and organs
  - Storage for calcium
  - movement of body
  - Bone marrow is the source of all blood cells
- Muscular system
  - Moves the bones
- Integumentary system
  - outer protective barrier
  - regulating body temperature
- Immune system
  - Defends against foreign invaders including cancers
  - prepare for replacing the injured cells

- Reproductive system
  - It is essential for perpetuating the species

Homoestatic control systems
I. Intrinsic (local) controls
- are inherent mechanisms within the organ
  - For example, **skeletal muscle** rapidly uses up $O_2 \rightarrow O_2$ decreases $\rightarrow$ act directly on the **smooth muscle** of the blood vessels $\rightarrow$ relaxation $\rightarrow$ the vessels dilate $\rightarrow$ blood flow increase $\rightarrow$ bringing more O_2

II. Extrinsic control is achieved by the **nervous** and **endocrine** systems
Mechanisms of extrinsic control
Negative feedback system (Fig. 58)
- Is the primary type of homeostatic control
- Opposes initial change
- When a **change** occur, the negative feedback will return it **back to normal**
- It have the following components
  1. Sensor
  2. Control center
  3. Effector: produces response

example
- When the **body temperature falls** the hypothalamus (via nerves) leads to
  - **Constriction of blood vessels of skin** $\rightarrow$ to conserve heat
  - Shivering of the skeletal muscles $\rightarrow$ to generate heat
  - **Hypothalamus** is the control center for temp control **(thermostat)**
  - $\rightarrow$ the temperature rises to normal
- When the **body temperature rise** above normal $\rightarrow$ **sweating** occur $\rightarrow$ it lowers the temperature to normal

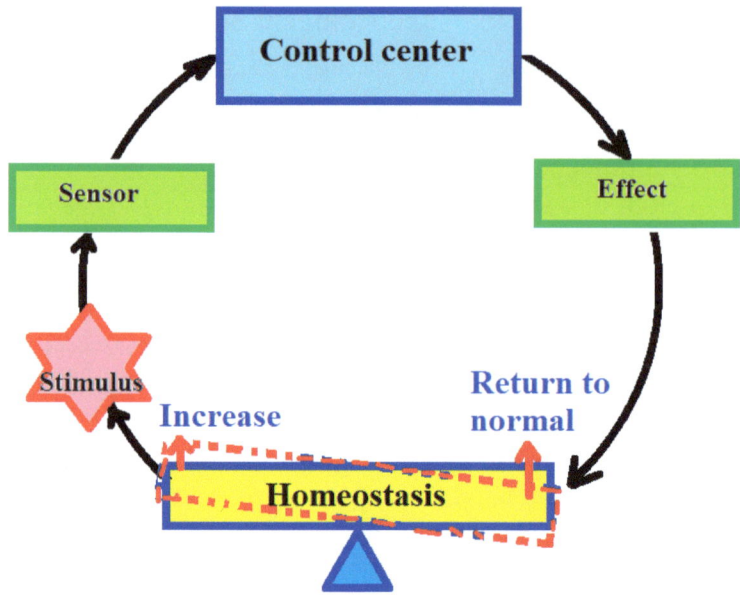

Figure 58: Homeostasis (negative feedback mechanism)

<u>**Factors homeostatically regulated include**</u>
1. Concentration of **nutrients**.
2. Concentration of **O2 and CO2.**
3. Concentration of **waste products**.
4. **pH**.
5. Concentrations of **water, salt, and other electrolytes.**
6. **Plasma volume & blood pressure.**
7. **Temperature**.

- <u>**Positive feedback system**</u>
  - Amplifies an initial change
  - It causes the initial stimulus to **continue to increase**
  - **Examples**: Blood clotting & the uterus in giving birth

Giving birth
  - The hormone **oxytocin** → powerful contractions of the uterus → push the baby against the cervix → **stretching of the cervix** → triggers the **release of more oxytocin** → and so on.
  - This **positive-feedback** cycle does not stop until the baby is born.

Chapter 2: Integumentary system

- **Integumentary system = Skin + appendages**
- **Skin appendages:**
  - Hair
  - Nails
  - Sweat glands
  - Sebaceous glands

Skin

Structure of the skin: 2 parts: epidermis + dermis

Epidermis
  - Keratinized stratified squamous epithelium
  - No blood vessels
  - Nutrients diffuse through tissue fluids

5 layers: (Fig. 1)
- **Stratum basale**: columnar cells, active in mitosis, produce keratinocytes, 10-25% are melanocytes
- **Stratum spinosum**: desmosomes appear as spines, contain prekeratin filaments (tension resisting)
- **Stratum granulosum**: cells flatten → have 2 types of granules:
  - **Keratohyaline granules**: → form part of keratin
  - **Lamellar granules**: are water resistant glycolipids, secreted extracellular
- **Stratum lucidum**: are flat dead keratinocytes, present only in thick skin (palm & sole)
- **Stratum corneum**: dead cells, forms ¾ of the epidermis thickness
  - **Keratin**: is formed by pre-keratin (intermediate filaments) + keratohyaline granules (act as glue)

- **Mnemonic:**
  - **Come** ⟶ Stratum **C**orneum
  - **Let's** ⟶ Stratum **L**ucidum
  - **Get** ⟶ Stratum **G**ranulosum
  - **Sun** ⟶ Stratum **S**pinosum
  - **Burn** ⟶ Stratum **B**asale

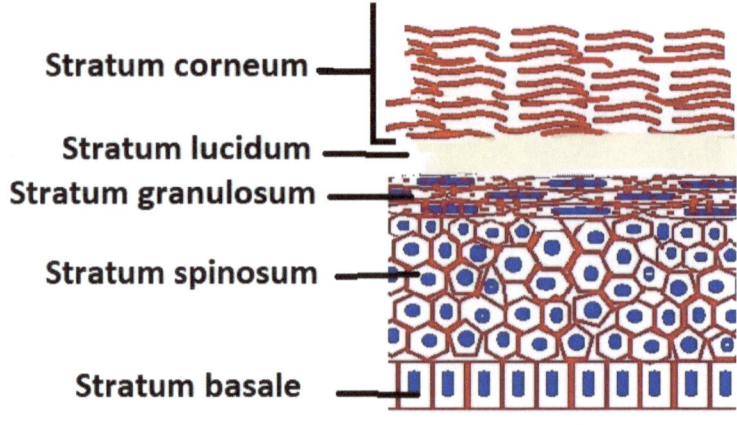

Stratum corneum

Stratum lucidum
Stratum granulosum

Stratum spinosum

Stratum basale

Figure 1: Layers of the epidermis of the skin

- <u>**Clinical notes:**</u> **Psoriasis** is an immune disorder → causes immune cells to target the epidermis → Increases the mitotic activity of the **epidermis**.

4 cell types
- **Keratinocytes**:
  - produced in the stratum basale
  - are connected together by desmosomes
  - produce keratin (protective for the skin)
  - die on reaching the surface
- **Melanocytes**: spider shaped cells → produce melanin in melanosomes (protect us from UV) → inject melanosomes into the keratinocytes
- **Langerhans cells**: star shaped, dendritic cells, formed in bone marrow, have immune function
- **Merkle cells**: receptors for touch

<u>**Dermis**</u>
- Dense connective tissue, have cells (fibroblasts + macrophages), with blood vessels, in matrix
- 2 layers: **(Fig. 2)**
  - **Papillary dermis**: loose areolar CT, have **dermal papillae**, forms epidermal ridges (= friction ridges), their pattern forms the finger prints
  - **Reticular dermis**: deeper, 80% of the thickness, network of collagen bundles which form the **cleavage lines**

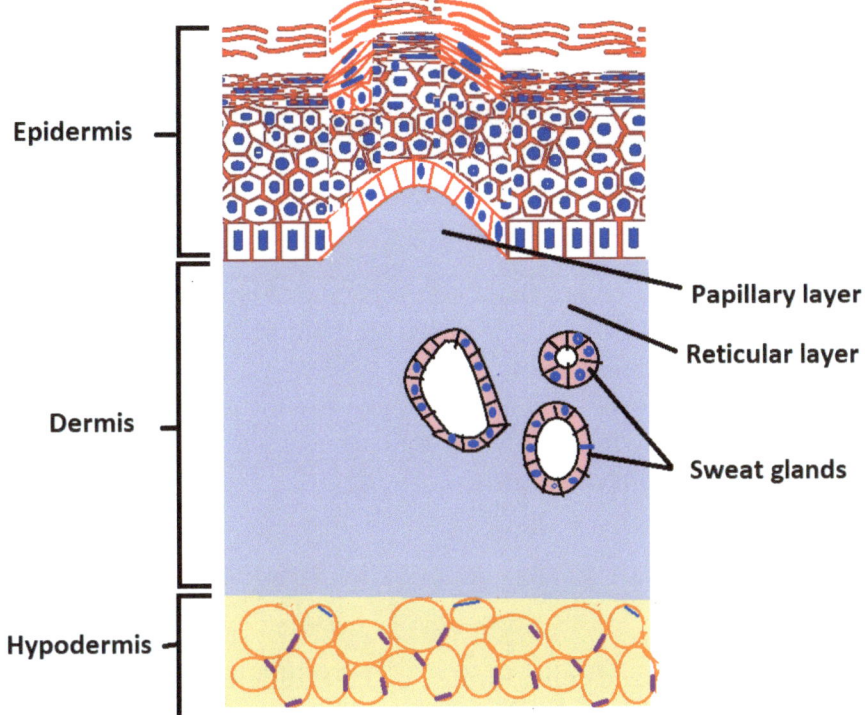

Figure 2: Skin and layers of the dermis

Clinical notes
- **incision** parallel to the **cleavage lines** gapes less & heals rapidly
- **striae** (white scars): is due to tearing of the dermis, as in pregnancy
- **blister**: is a pocket of fluid between dermis & epidermis
- diminished blood flow to the dermis → causes **ulcers**, as in **bed sores**

Hypodermis
- = **Subcutaneous tissue** = **superficial fascia**, mostly adipose tissue, is not part of the skin

Skin color
- is determined by **melanin**
- ranges from yellow to black
- formed by **melanocytes** from tyrosine by **tyrosinase enzyme** → produce melanin in melanosomes → are injected into keratinocytes
- all people have the same number of melanocytes

- **Black people** have more melanosomes → dark skin → to protect DNA of their skin from UV of the sun.
- **Tanning**: darkening of the skin due to increase melanin synthesis
- **Carotine**: yellow/ orange pigment, in stratum corneum
- **Albinism**: lack of melanin pigment which affect all the body
- **Vitiligo**: regional defects in melanocyte function

Alteration of skin color
- **Cyanosis**: blue color due to unoxygenated blood
- **Pallor**: low BP or anemia or reduced blood flow to dermal vessels
- **Blushing**: red skin, as in fever
- **Jaundice**: yellow skin or sclera, due to bilirubin
- **Bruises** (ecchymosis): red, purple, green, yellow color of the skin as the hematoma is absorbed

Hair

Structure of hair
- Dead keratinized cells, formed by hair follicles
- 2 parts:
    - **shaft** (rounded thread, silky if it is perfectly round)
    - **root** (present inside the **hair follicle**)
- **Consists of 3 keratinized concentric layers: (Fig. 3)**
    - **Medulla**: soft keratin, absent in fine hairs
    - **Cortex**: several layers of flat cells
    - **Cuticle**: outermost heavily keratinized layer, it wears away from the tip of hair

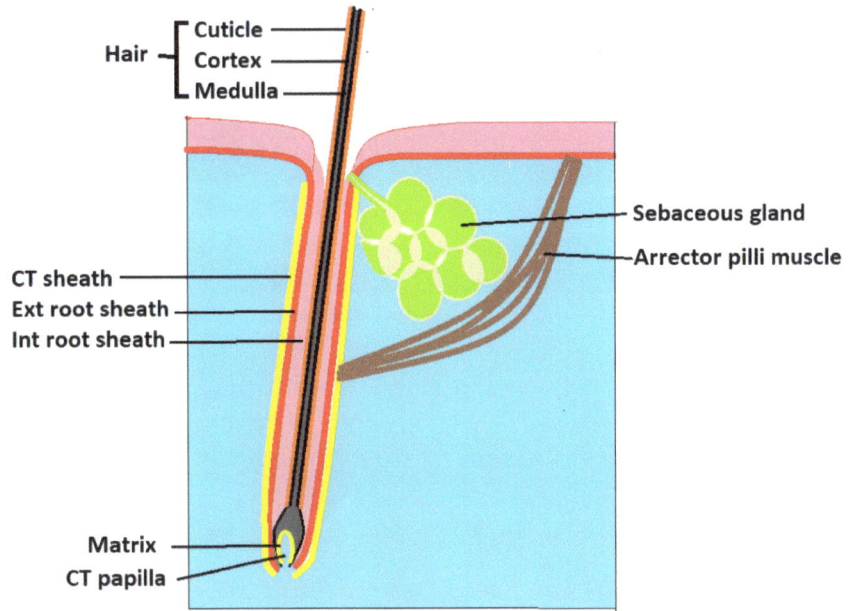

Figure 3: Structure of the hair

Hair follicle
- Downward folding of epidermis into the dermis
- Its wall has 3 layers **(Fig. 3)**:
    1. **Fibrous sheath** of CT, derived from dermis
    2. **External root sheath**: continuation of epidermis
    3. **Internal root sheath**: derived from matrix cells
- **Hair bulb:** expanded deep end of the hair follicle
    - Is surrounded with receptor nerve plexus (sense bending)
- **Hair papilla**: protrude into the bulb, contain capillaries for nutrition & growth of hair
- **Hair matrix cells**: lines the hair papilla, divide rapidly → produce hair cells

Arrector pilli muscle:
- it pulls the hair upright and dimples the skin → produce **goose bumps** in response to cold or fear.
- It forces sebum out to lubricate skin.

Hair types
- **Vellus hair**: pale, fine hairs, in children & female body
- **Terminal hair**: darker, stimulated by androgens (testosterone)

Hair growth:

- **Growth cycle of hair follicle**:
  - active growth phase (4 years)
  - resting phase (shedding occur)
  - The cycle occur asynchronous
- Average growth 2 mm/ W

Clinical notes:
- **Hirsutism**: coarse terminal hairs in female,
  - Occur in polycystic ovary syndrome or adrenal tumors
- **Baldness**: by age 60Y, terminal hairs are replaced with vellus hairs, male baldness is genetically determined
- **Telogen effluvium (TE)**: synchronous growth cycle, occur after surgery, shock or emotional stress

Nails
- Consist of hard keratin
- Has **root** (embedded in skin), **body** (nail plate), **free edge (Fig. 4)**

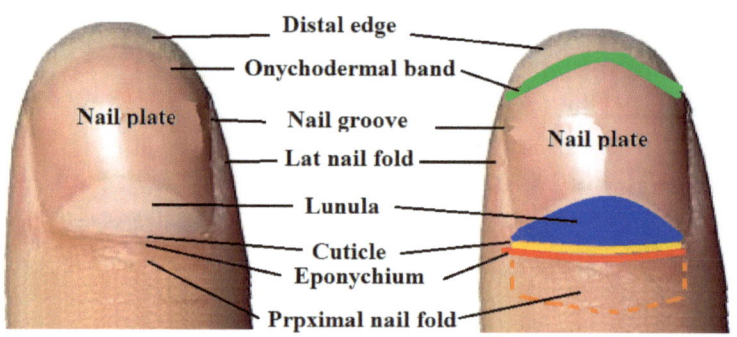

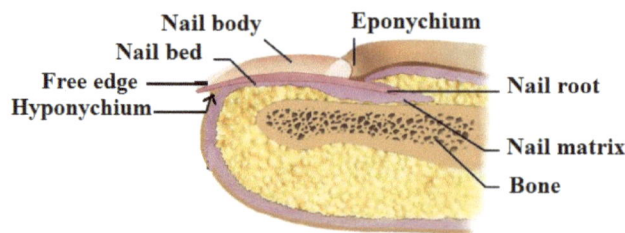

Figure 4: Structure of the nail

Nail bed:
- corresponds to the deep layers of epidermis
- appears pink (rich in capillaries)

Nail matrix:
- is its thickened proximal part
- responsible for **nail growth**
- White **lunule** appears over it

Nail fold:
- the lateral & proximal borders
- **Eponychium**: the proximal fold

Hyponychium:
- space under the distal end

Koilonychia:
- concave nail, signals iron deficiency

Skin glands

Sebaceous glands (Fig. 5)
- Simple branched alveolar gland
- Found all over the body, except palm & sole
- central cells accumulate oil until burst (**holocrine** gland) →
  secreted as **sebum** (lubricates hair & skin + bactericidal effect)
- Secrete into hair follicle by arrector pilli contraction
- Activity increases during puberty, under male sex hormones

Clinical notes

Acne: active inflammation of the sebaceous glands, due to:
- – Accumulation of **sebum**
- – Infection with Propionibacterium acne

Seborrhea: overactive sebaceous glands → with fast flowing **sebum** →
slough off oily **scales**

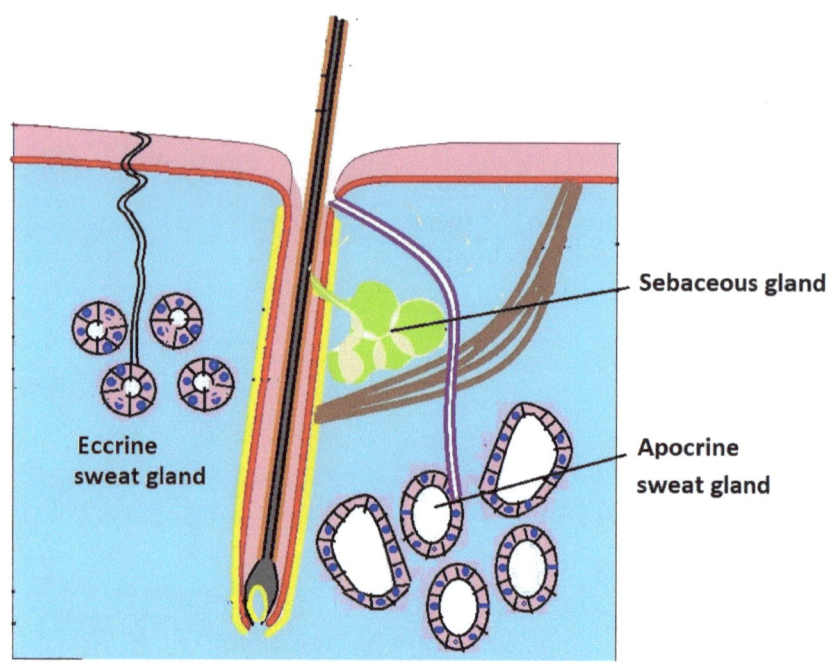

Figure 5: Glands of the skin

Sweat glans

- Present everywhere, except nipple & part of ext genitalia
- Secretory cells, surrounded by myoepithelial cells → contract to squeeze the secretions
- Supplied by autonomic nerves
- 2 types: **(Fig. 5)**

Eccrine (merocrine):

- all over the body, abundant in palm, sole & forehead
- simple, coiled tubular gland present in dermis
- duct opens into the surface of the **skin**
- secrete **sweat: hypotonic** secretion released from blood by exocytosis, **acidic** pH 4-6
- prevent overheating

Apocrine:

- Present in axilla & anogenital areas
- Larger, deeper than eccrine
- Duct opens into **hair follicle**
- Secretion: are **vicious**, similar to eccrine + fatty & protein material
- Bacteria decompose its organic material giving **body odor**
- Start functioning at puberty, **under effect of androgens**
- Function: may act as **pheromones** (sexual attraction)

- Modified apocrine glands:
  - **Ceruminous glands:** in ext ear, secrete cerumen = ear wax
  - **Mammary glands:** produce milk only after childbirth.

Functions of the skin
- **Protection**:
  - Physical barrier: keratinized cells
  - Chemical barrier: acid secretion + melanin (prevent UV)
  - biological barriers: dendritic cells (triggers immune response) & dermal macrophages (engulf viruses & bacteria)
- Regulation of body **temperature**:
  - evaporation of sweat
  - Blood vessels: VD in case of heat, VC in case of cold
- Cutaneous **sensation**: Meissner's corpuscles (touch), Pacinian corpuscle (pressure), free N endings (pain), hair follicles (touch)
- Metabolic functions: sunrays convert cholesterol into **vitamin D precursor** ($\rightarrow$ Ca^{++} absorption)
- **Blood reservoir**: 5% of blood
- Excretion of water & salts in **sweat**

Disorders of the skin
- **Athlete's foot** is caused by **fungal** infection of the skin of the toes and sole.
- **Impetigo** is caused by a **bacterial** infection that results in pustules with crust over it.
- **Candidiasis** is caused by a **yeast** infection, affecting the diaper area in infants.
- **Eczema:** an **inflammation** caused by sensitivity to various chemicals (e.g., soap or detergents), to certain fabrics, or even to heat or dryness.
- **Dandruff:** is caused by an accelerated rate of **keratinization** in certain areas of the scalp, producing flaking and itching.
- **Urticaria:** is an **allergic** reaction characterized by reddish, elevated patches and itching.

Skin Cancer
Basal cell carcinoma
- Begins in the basal cell layer

- It is triggered by UV radiation + suppressing the immune system → its cells can not detect the tumor.
- The signs: **open sore**, recurring reddish circular patch with raised edge.

Squamous cell carcinoma
- begins in the superficial cells
- It is triggered by excessive UV exposure.
- The signs are the same as basal cell carcinoma, except that it may give **wart-like** or scaly growth that bleeds, but refuses to heal.

Malignant melanoma
- starts in the **melanocytes**
- It looks like an unusual mole of a **spilled ink spot**, which can also itch, hurt, or feel numb.
- Usually due to sun exposure.

Kaposi's sarcoma
- Skin cancer, seen in patients with **AIDS**, and in patients with weak immune system.
- appears as red, blue, or black **spots** on the skin.
- responds to the treatment of "AIDS"

Raised growths on the skin, can be:
- **Moles** are due to an overgrowth of melanocytes
- **Warts** are due to a viral infection.

Wound Healing
- A **wound** will be filled with **blood** → give **clot**.
- Inflammatory chemicals → draw **WBCs** + **fibroblasts** → pull the margins of the wound together → **proliferate** → **scar**
- The basal layer of the **epidermis** proliferates → **close the wound**

Surface lesions of the skin (Fig. 6)
- **Erythema** = redness of the skin.
- **Macule** = a spot that is neither raised nor depressed and is less than 1 cm in size, as in measles
    - **Patch** = A flat lesion greater than 1 cm.
- **Papule** = pimple: a firm, raised area less than 1 cm in size, as in chickenpox and in the second stage of syphilis
    - **nodule** = solid, raised, and round lesion larger than 1 cm

- **Vesicle** a small fluid-filled sac less than 5 mm in size, as in chickenpox
    - **bulla** = similar lesion greater than 5 mm in size
- **Pustule:** a pus-filled lesion of less than 1 cm.

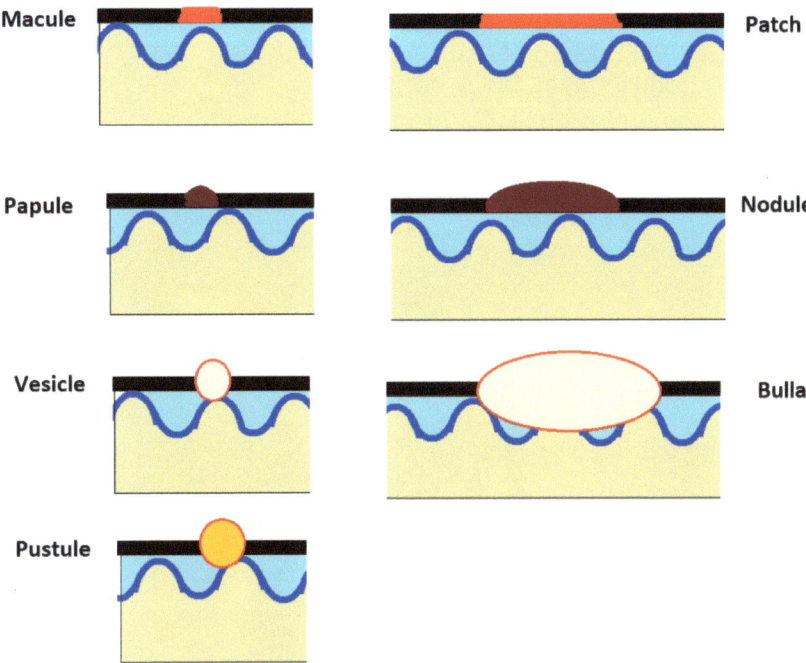

Figure 6 Surface lesions of the skin

Deep lesions of the skin

- **Excoriation** = a scratch into the skin.
- **Laceration** = a wound made by tearing of the skin.
- **Ulcer** = a sore associated with disintegration and death of skin.
    - **Pressure ulcers** = appear where the bony projections rests on skin, such as the spine, heel, elbow, or hip.
- **Fissure** = a crack in the skin.
    - As in athlete's foot

Burns

- Burns are skin injuries caused by heat, radioactive, chemical, and electrical agents.
- The severity is estimated by the "**rule of nines**" **(Fig. 7)**
- It divides the body into regions:
    - the head and neck, 9%

- each upper limb, 9%;
- each lower limb, 2x9%
- the front and back portions of the trunk, 2x9% each
- the perineum, which includes the anal and urogenital regions, 1%

A burn is considered critical injury if it is a
(1) 2nd degree burn covering **25%** or more
(2) 3rd degree burn covering **10%** or more of the body
(3) **3rd degree** burn on the **face, hands or feet**.
(4) 4th degree burn of any part of the body

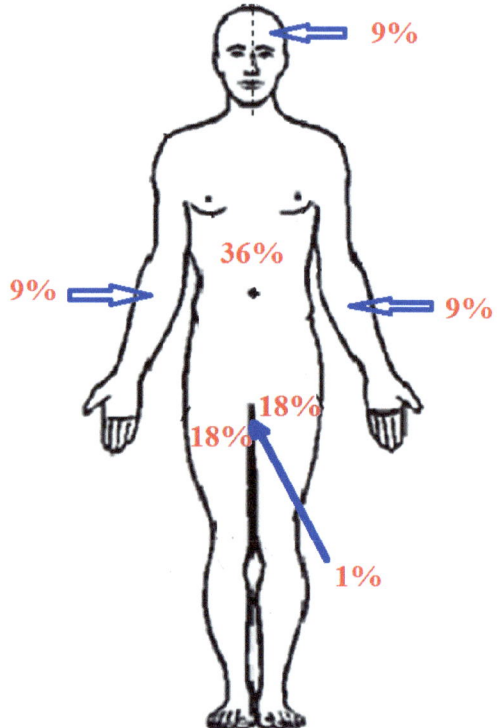

9%

9%

36%

9%

18%

18%

1%

Figure 7: Burns- the rule of nines

Degrees:
- **1st degree**
  - Affects the **epidermis** only
  - redness and pain
  - The damaged skin peels off in about a week.
  - Treatment is the management of pain.
- **2nd degree**
  - Affects the **epidermis + part of the dermis**.
  - Redness, pain, blistering.

82

- – Heals in 14 days with little scarring.
- **3rd degree**
  - – Destroys the **entire thickness of the skin**.
  - – The surface of the wound is leathery, brown or black.
  - – Destroys pain receptors, blood vessels, sweat glands, sebaceous glands, and hair follicles.
- **4th degree**
  - – Involves skin + tissues **down to the bone**.
  - – It is mostly fatal

Effect of aging

- **Skin** is loose & wrinkled, due to loose attachment to the underlying tissues
- **Epidermis** maintains its thickness.
- **Dermis** becomes thinner, with less collagen & less elastic.
- **Hypodermis** Adipose tissue of the face and hands decreases → gives cold hands → bruise easily
- **Blood vessels & sweat glands** became few → limited homeostatic adjustment to heat
- **Hair follicles & sebaceous glands** decrease in number → cracking of the skin
- **Melanocytes** decrease in number → gray hair & pale skin.
- Ultraviolet radiation of the sun → pigmented patches of skin.

Skin Homeostasis

Skin helps the following systems:
- **Lymphatic** system in protecting all body systems.
- **Kidney**: in regulating water balance and waste excretion by sweating
- **skeletal system** in storing calcium by producing vitamin D upon exposed to UV
- **muscular system** by regulating body temperature (by VC & VD of the blood vessels & by sweat glands)
- **Nervous system** by receptors, which carry sensory information from the external environment.
- Skin responds to **endocrine hormones**
  - – **Androgens** stimulate hair growth and sebaceous gland secretion
  - – **estrogens** stimulate fat deposition

Appendix 1: Learning objectives

Anatomical terminology
1. Define the following anatomical terms of position: Anterior/ventral, posterior/dorsal, superior, inferior, medial, median, lateral, proximal, distal, superficial, deep, prone, supine, palmar & plantar.
2. Describe the following anatomical planes: transverse/horizontal, sagittal/vertical plane and the coronal/frontal plane.
3. Define and demonstrate the terms used to describe movement: Flexion, extension, abduction, adduction, medial rotation, lateral rotation, inversion, eversion, supination, pronation, plantar-flexion, dorsi-flexion, and circumduction.
4. Compare and contrast the systematic changes associated with growth and ageing in children, adults and the elderly.
5. Identify the major surface and bony landmarks in each body region (e.g. occipital protuberance, orbital ridge, nasal bones, mastoid process, cervical to sacro-coccygeal vertebrae and associated joints, shoulder girdle and upper limb, sternal region, ribs and costal margin, pelvic girdle and lower limb).

Histological overview
6. Identify and describe the components of the basic cell.
7. Identify and describe the features of the epithelial tissues (simple squamous, stratified squamous, transitional, cuboidal, columnar and ciliated).
8. Identify and describe the general structure of a neuron.
9. Describe and contrast different types of cartilage (hyaline, fibrocartilage and elastic cartilage).
10. Compare and contrast the structural features of skeletal, smooth and cardiac muscle.
11. Describe the role of the types of connective tissues.

Integumentary system
12. Describe the epidermis, dermis & subcutaneous layers of the skin and appendages (hair follicles, sweat glands, nails).
13. Describe the main diseases affecting the skin, including the burns.

Appendix 2: Bibliography

1. Connolly et al.: Core anatomy syllabus for Undergraduate Nursing. *Journal of Anatomy*, 2018, 232: 721-728, published by John Wiley & Sons Ltd.
2. Elain Marieb and Katja Hoehn: Human Anatomy & Physiology, 11th edition. 2010, Pearson.
3. Lauralee Sherwood: Fundamentals of Human Physiology, 4th edition. 2011, Brooks/Cole, USA
4. Gerard J. Tortora And Bryan Derrickson: Principles of Anatomy and Physiology, 14th Edition, 2014 John Wiley and Sons, USA.
5. Memmler's the Human Body in Health in Disease Author: Cohen, Wood, and Memmler Publisher: Lippincott Williams & Wilkins Year: 2018 ISBN: 978-1496380500
6. Gray's Basic Anatomy, Richard Drake, Wayne Vogl, and Adam W. M.□, 2nd Edition, Elsevier Philadephia, 2017.
7. Mader S, Windelspecht M. Human Biology. 13th Edition. McGraw-Hill Science/Engineering/Math. 2013
8. Young B, Lowe J, Stevens A, Heath J, Deakin P. Wheater's Functional Histology: A Text and Colour Atlas. 6th Edition. Churchill Livingstone.2013.
9. John E. Hall. Guyton & Hall Text Book of Medical Physiology. 13th Edn. Elsevier Philadephia, 2016.
10. Koeppen, & Stanton. Berne & Levy Physiology. 7th Edition, Elsevier. 2018.
11. Barrett K, Barman S, Boitano S, Brooks H. Ganong's Review of Medical Physiology. 26th Edition. LANGE Basic Science. 2019
12. Human embryology Keith. L. Moore 5th edition.

Appendix 3: Human A&P Booklets

The following parts are available as **e-booklets**:

- Part 1/7: Introduction to A & P + Integumentary system
- Part 2/7: Skeletal and Muscular systems
- Part 3/7: Cardiovascular system and Blood
- Part 4/7: Respiratory and Immune systems
- Part 5/7: Digestive and Endocrine systems
- Part 6/7: Urinary and Reproductive systems
- Part 7/7: CNS & Special Senses

The 7 parts will be compiled and published as a single **paper booklet**.